A WOMAN'S GUIDE TO
CANNABIS

A WOMAN'S GUIDE TO
CANNABIS

Using Marijuana *to* Feel Better, Look Better,
Sleep Better—*and Get High Like a Lady*

NIKKI FURRER

WORKMAN PUBLISHING
NEW YORK

For Joey

Library of Congress Cataloging-in-Publication Data is available.

ISBN 978-1-5235-0200-4

Design by Becky Terhune
Cover and interior illustrations by Lisel Ashlock

Workman books are available at special discounts when purchased in bulk for premiums and sales promotions as well as for fund-raising or educational use. Special editions or book excerpts can also be created to specification. For details, contact the Special Sales Director at the address below, or send an email to specialmarkets@workman.com.

Workman Publishing Co., Inc.
225 Varick Street
New York, NY 10014-4381
workman.com

WORKMAN is a registered trademark of Workman Publishing Co., Inc.

Printed in China
First printing November 2018

10 9 8 7 6 5 4 3 2

All names of people used in anecdotes are pseudonyms, with the exception of the author's mother.

CONTENTS

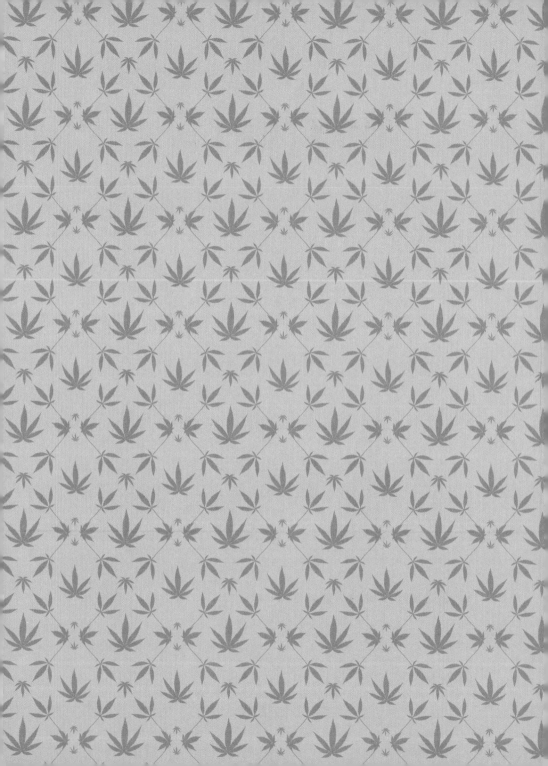

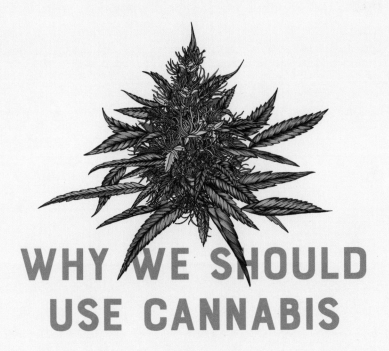

Part One

WHY WE SHOULD USE CANNABIS

Before I began working in the legal marijuana industry, I owned an independent bookstore. It was fun and sometimes thrilling, and many book lovers have the same fantasy: "Oh, I'd love to own a bookstore. I would just curl up and read. All. The. Time." But the reality is that bookstore owners don't have time to read, because they're too stressed out about keeping customers and paying bills.

During the last, awful week before the doors of my little shop closed forever, I used a gift card for a much-needed massage. "Relax your shoulders, please," the massage therapist told me. I took a deep breath and tried. "You have the most tension I've ever felt in a person," said the massage therapist, and I burst into tears.

So when I was ready to begin my post-bookstore career, I knew I didn't want stress. I wanted to continue helping people—matching a reader to the exact book they're craving is a magical experience—but I had to think about my own health, too. So, like hundreds of other marijuana migrants, I packed everything I owned into a U-Haul and moved to Colorado, where I learned how to grow thousands of marijuana plants at a time. I stood behind the counter at dispensaries and spoke with hundreds of medical marijuana patients about their cannabis use. I began working in other states, building brand-new marijuana dispensaries and cultivation centers, creating new strains of marijuana, as well as new edible and topical products. Now, I'm working as hard as ever, but my shoulders are relaxed, my back doesn't hurt, and my depression is a distant memory.

Now that I'm in my forties, cannabis makes me feel prettier and more relaxed than I ever was in my twenties or thirties.

Even after a car accident fractured my spine and created permanent back pain, medical marijuana makes me healthier and happier than I've ever been before.

In dispensaries, we answer the same beginner questions over and over again: "How do I use a vape pen?" "Will I get high from this cream?" "Can I give this to my dog?" I'm still a bookseller at heart, and I didn't have a book to recommend to new cannabis patients. Sure, there are lots of books about marijuana—cookbooks and gardening books and books about the history of marijuana legalization—but I couldn't find a book that could take my mother through her first shopping trip at the dispensary and her first time getting high.

Because the more we know about cannabis, the easier it is to use it in a way that's effective for us. So I wrote this book for anyone who wants to feel better, look better, and sleep better. Everything we teach new patients at the dispensary is in these pages, including how cannabis works, why it works, and how to make marijuana gummies at home. Plus there are a few surprises in this book that you won't learn at the dispensary.

We don't hang a "No Boys Allowed" sign on our ladies' cannabis clubhouse door. Men are more than welcome to read this book, too. Cannabis is for everyone.

WHAT CANNABIS OFFERS

"Nikki, can you come out here?" My twentysomething, rainbow-haired coworker opened the door to the garden and yelled over the music.

"On my way," I yelled back. I set down my clippers, pulled off my gloves, and left behind the marijuana plant I was cutting up. In the waiting room of the dispensary, I found a well-dressed woman in her late sixties. A cane leaned against the coffee table that held a neat pile of new-patient paperwork. A younger woman sat next to her on the couch, dressed in the ubiquitous style of Denver—casual hiking gear.

"Hi," I said. I flashed my customer service smile as I approached them. "What can I help you with today?"

The older woman looked up. When she saw a forty-year-old woman in yoga pants and glasses, she visibly relaxed. "My daughter talked me into this. She helped me get the card. I have trouble sleeping and pain in my hip from the surgery, and . . . she said it would help, but I don't know where to start. I've never smoked anything. . . ." Her voice faded and she waved a helpless hand over the paperwork.

"You know, I was just reading a study about baby boomers who smoked pot occasionally in the sixties. It seems they don't get diagnosed with Alzheimer's at the rate that nonsmokers do," I said. "Marijuana can prevent symptoms of dementia, even decades later." I smiled at her, waiting for the inevitable response.

There it was: Her eyes lit up and she smiled to herself. "Really?" she whispered.

"Mom!" The younger woman laughed.

"Somebody's pants are on fire," I said.

"Well . . ." The older woman smiled at her daughter. "It was just a few times. In college. In the sorority house. We knew it was wrong."

"A plant that makes us happier and healthier isn't wrong," I said.

We talked for an hour. Cannabinoids, modes of administration, dosing. On the coffee table, I lined up gummies, creams, and transdermal patches. We practiced a breathing meditation she could use to relax if her first dose caused any anxiety. She decided on a sucker and a salve for her hip. I gave her my cell phone number and told her to call if she had any problems.

You might even consider cannabis a superfood.

She called the dispensary the next day.

"I slept through the night," she said, and I could hear the smile in her voice. "And I walked to the mailbox without my cane. Maybe we weren't so wrong, back at the sorority."

The sorority girls weren't wrong at all. After decades of reefer madness propaganda, we're now learning about how good this demonized plant is for our health and happiness. Cannabis doesn't just make us feel high and happy; it also has powerful analgesic, anti-inflammatory, antioxidant, antibacterial, antifungal, antianxiety, and antidepressant qualities.

The marijuana plant has lots of different ways to make us happy, healthy, and beautiful. We might even consider it a superfood. We eat well and exercise for healthy bodies, and a daily dose of cannabis in the right amount can be just as effective for keeping us happy and healthy.

More than half of all Americans have access to legal medical marijuana, and more states are creating new medical marijuana laws every year, which means more and more Americans are starting to use cannabis to cure what ails them, and in states where people use legal marijuana, rates of opioid overdoses drop by 25 percent.*

Many people know someone who indulges in the "mommy cocktail"—a glass of wine and a Xanax—to relax, but mixing pills and booze is a lethal threat, especially for women over forty. Alcohol and prescription pills are legal, socially acceptable, easily obtained, and paid for by health insurance. Women are drinking more alcohol than ever before, and when we combine that with the fact that prescription pills are handed out like candy, it's not surprising that the opioid epidemic has hit every suburb in the country.

Prescriptions like opioids, sleeping pills, antidepressants, and antianxiety pills have more side effects than the symptoms they relieve. The pill that reduces a bit of pain also causes insomnia, so now there's a sleeping pill. The sleeping pill works too well, so a stimulant is prescribed. That pill causes anxiety, so now there's a stash of Xanax in the medicine cabinet. And when those pills stop working we take more, so now there's another doctor and another prescription pad. A year later, the

*Marcus A. Bachhuber, MD, Brendan Saloner, PhD, Chinazo O. Cunningham, MD, and Colleen L. Barry, PhD, "Medical Cannabis Laws and Opioid Analgesic Overdose Mortality in the United States, 1999–2010," *JAMA Internal Medicine* 174, no. 10 (October 2014): 1668–1673.

pills don't work as well, which leads to stronger drugs to relieve the original source of pain. Swapping out the medicine cabinet for marijuana can prevent that downward spiral to rehab.

My mother's seventysomething, conservative, midwestern friends are fascinated with marijuana, and they ask a lot of questions.

"Will it help my Parkinson's?"

"What about arthritis?"

"Will I gain weight?"

"Am I going to turn into a Democrat?"

"Is it like I remember?"

My mom's neighbor spotted me when I was visiting and ran outside to talk about topical creams for her arthritic hands. Her son the lawyer had brought her a cream from Seattle. It worked so well and she needed more and did I happen to have any?

"I don't think I should sell drugs in my mom's backyard," I said. "I'm middle aged, but my mom will still get really mad."

"It's not drugs. It's a miracle." She smiled and waved both hands at me.

It's not just ladies of a certain age who are using cannabis. Ladies of *all* ages are using cannabis to get high, feel better, and look better. My fortysomething friends have just as many questions as my mother's friends, because the marijuana in dispensaries today is so different from the marijuana we remember from our youth.

REALISTIC EXPECTATIONS

Legal cannabis is curative and restorative. It makes us sleep better, eat better, and feel better. But it's important to have realistic expectations, so no, I will not tell you that cannabis cures cancer. I have seen many patients make miraculous strides in their cancer treatments when they incorporate cannabis with chemotherapy and other oncologist-recommended treatments. I've seen scans the Mayo Clinic can't explain—with cancer having just disappeared.

But I've also been to a lot of funerals. The success I've seen is always with stage 1 or stage 2 cancer; never once have I seen cannabis completely cure anyone with stage 3 or 4 cancer.

Cannabis is the only medicine I take, but it doesn't work by itself. I still need to do yoga and move my body through its entire range of motion to keep everything healthy and pain-free, and I still need to meditate on a daily basis to reduce stress and anxiety. Using cannabis makes it easier for me to do the things I need to do to get and stay healthy, because getting high and doing yoga and meditation feels amazing. Food and water taste better, so I eat healthier, and beauty sleep comes more easily. But even with cannabis medicine, we still have to do everything we can to take care of ourselves.

I'm a lawyer, not a doctor, but after years of reading medical research on cannabis, I firmly believe that many people would benefit from a small, daily, preventative dose of cannabis. Just a little bit every day is enough to reduce inflammation, anxiety, depression, stress, and pain, slow the onset of demen-tia and other signs of aging, and boost our mood. Cannabis has replaced antidepressants, antianxiety medication, and pain prescriptions for many people I know. But let me be perfectly clear: I am not suggesting you change any medication unless you discuss it with your doctor.

MDS AND MEDICAL MARIJUANA

If we ask five different doctors what they think about medical marijuana, we will get five different opinions in response. Some doctors are wildly opposed, many doctors think it's pretty harmless and also not really medicine, some claim they haven't researched cannabis enough to know what to believe, and some doctors have seen positive results and actively encourage their patients to use cannabis. Everyone agrees that more research needs to be done so we can fully understand how the cannabis plant can be used to make us feel better, but some doctors are more willing to experiment with what we know now.

Specialists in cancer, pain management, and neurolog-ical issues tend to be more supportive of cannabis, simply because they have seen improvement in their own patients. "My oncologist told me to ask my kids to get marijuana for me" is something I've heard more than once. Pain management doctors—the ones who write most of the opioid prescriptions—are usually the first doctors to sign off on medical marijuana recommendations. Pediatricians are always opposed to marijuana because they have a legitimate concern with wanting to keep kids and teenagers from using it recreationally. There is an age issue here, as well—older doctors, no matter what their specialty, tend to be less supportive of cannabis than younger doctors.

Don't be afraid to talk to your doctor or your parent's doctor about cannabis. Most likely, other patients have already asked them about it and they have an answer ready. Or they might want to do a little research on their own. In the "Suggested Reading List" section of this book, I've listed several books written by doctors who have studied the latest cannabis research.

Don't feel discouraged if your primary care or specialist physicians aren't as supportive as you want them to be. Don't be surprised if you've spent more time researching cannabis than they have. Medical schools do not teach cannabis medicine, so this is a new subject for doctors, too.

Unfortunately, even if your doctor approves of cannabis use, she still may be constrained from signing the recommendation form. Doctors have employers' and medical malpractice insurance, and they can only do what they are allowed to do. Hospitals and insurance companies are nervous about the federal restrictions against cannabis, and to avoid any legal risk, they often tell doctors not to sign off on marijuana.

My brother's neurologist was okay with trying cannabis for his seizures, but he refused to sign for the card because he was leaving the country for an extended period of time and wouldn't be there to supervise the cannabis experiment. Disappointing for us, but an understandable concern for the doctor.

If your regular doctor won't sign the recommendation for cannabis, go to a doctor who will. In each state there are doctors who specialize in cannabis recommendations. These doctors and their staff know what is necessary in your state—a certain diagnosis, fingerprints, and residency requirements—so check to see if there is one in your area by calling your local dispensary. They will be able to guide you to a doctor.

Every state has doctors who specialize in cannabis.

Some states make it easier to get a patient card, and some make it as difficult as possible. In Colorado, I saw a doctor who barely looked up from his notes, and his assistant put everything together for me. I just waved at my back and said "car accident." He signed off on my paperwork and I was buying weed within an hour. In Illinois, it took two months of research, networking, phone calls, and appointments to find a doctor who would sign the certification. Then I had to make an eight-hour road trip, get blood work done, get fingerprinted for a background check, and wait more than a month for my card to arrive in the mail.

In every state, the doctor signs a recommendation (or, as in Illinois, a certification of the qualifying condition), not a prescription. There isn't enough medical research yet to know how to treat specific conditions and pain with specific doses and products, so most doctors do not know how much, or what kind, of cannabis is best for you. That's why they sign a recommendation rather than a prescription. It means they know marijuana will help that patient find relief from their symptoms and conditions, but they aren't giving a specific dosage.

Each state has its own list of qualifying conditions that are allowed to be treated with cannabis. Some states with new marijuana programs have a very limited list of debilitating conditions and diseases that qualify. Some states allow arthritis and post-traumatic stress disorder (PTSD) patients to use cannabis; some allow Parkinson's and cerebral palsy patients to do so. Some states, especially those with older, more mature marijuana laws, allow a card for all kinds of reasons, including depression and anxiety. The top dozen that usually make the list are cancer, HIV/AIDS, seizures/epilepsy, glaucoma, multiple sclerosis (MS)/muscle spasms, Crohn's disease, severe nausea/wasting syndrome, Parkinson's disease, anything terminal, amyotrophic lateral sclerosis (ALS), Alzheimer's disease, and chronic pain. The majority of patients qualify for a card with a diagnosis of chronic pain, because it is such a catchall diagnosis. In Colorado, I got a medical card for chronic pain, and so did every twentysomething I met in the cannabis industry. But in Illinois, I had to get a diagnosis of fibromyalgia to qualify for a card so I could treat my sciatic nerve pain, because chronic and sciatic nerve pain are not on the list.

There's no rhyme or reason to the lists of qualifying conditions, other than pure politics. These lists are haggled over and negotiated between politicians and desperate patients testifying at hearings. Hopefully, as we continue to research cannabis, these restrictions will lift and anyone will be able to use cannabis for any reason. Until then, we all have to jump through the hoops they put in front of us.

Unfortunately, the one hoop we don't have to worry about with medical marijuana is health insurance. Health insurance won't pay for the doctor visit to get the card, it won't pay for the card, and it won't pay for your medicine. New medical marijuana patients, who are used to paying a few dollars for a month's supply of pharmacy painkillers, may find themselves spending several hundreds of dollars in cash at the dispensary every month.

I believe proper, effective cannabis medicine will be manufactured by pharmaceutical companies, available at any pharmacy, and covered by health insurance plans. That day is at least fifteen years away. Once federal restrictions against cannabis are lifted, life will be easier and less painful—but when you're waiting on the federal government to act, you need to be very, very patient.

CANNABIS FOR PAIN RELIEF

When Karen came to the dispensary for the first time, her husband pushed her in a wheelchair. She had a bag in her lap, full of prescription medications for pain and depression. Karen could barely walk, and when she did, she winced in pain. She couldn't work anymore, she couldn't exercise, and she couldn't babysit her grandchildren. Her husband had retired and they wanted to travel and see the world, but Karen barely had the strength to pull a suitcase through the airport.

Her diagnosis was vague because doctors couldn't find the source of her pain. Three different specialists wrote prescriptions for her on a regular basis, and Karen had the flat affect and tone of someone taking too many pills. Some days, she was a little groggy. Other days, she seemed distracted and irritated, and she was never, ever, nice. To anyone. She barked nothing but instructions and demands at her husband, who seemed just as miserable as she was. Once a week they stopped by the dispensary to buy more gummy candies and pain cream. The budtenders encouraged Karen's husband to try some candy himself, but he always refused.

After a month of marijuana use, Karen smiled at me when I made a joke. She didn't laugh, but she did give a real smile. Two weeks later, she and her husband walked into the dispensary without a wheelchair. This time, they were both smiling.

Two months after her first marijuana candy, Karen was babysitting her grandchildren again, two days a week. She started taking walks around the block after dinner. Her doctors acknowledged that she had less pain and lowered her prescription dosages. She started going to her book club again and making plans with her friends. Her husband surprised her with a trip to New York and tickets to see the musical *Hamilton*.

"Hi, honey! You look so nice today. That's the perfect blue for your coloring," Karen said to me one day at the dispensary. Her tone was friendly and warm, and it was like meeting a whole new person. She looked taller and prettier and fifteen years younger.

Her husband noticed me noticing Karen. She moved down the counter to look at some new edibles, and he leaned over to whisper. "Thank you," he said. "This marijuana stuff has changed our lives. I don't know what we'd do without it." He patted my hand and went to join his wife.

Most of the people who walk into a dispensary are there because they have pain. Back pain. Arthritis. Fibromyalgia. Menstrual cramps. Plantar fasciitis. Sciatic nerve pain. Sprains, tears, and breaks. Some pain throbs, some aches, and some burns. Pain can be debilitating to our quality of life. Pain slows us down and holds us back, and if we try to reduce it with a prescription, the side effects may make it worse—or even kill us.

Cannabis is a strong analgesic, which means it relieves pain, but it is also a powerful anti-inflammatory. Pain as a result of inflammation responds well to small doses of cannabis.

Cannabis is not a miracle cure, but I've met hundreds of medical marijuana patients who are able to function because cannabis reduced their pain when nothing else worked. There are negative side effects to cannabis—short-term memory loss,

Cannabis is a strong analgesic, which means it relieves pain.

anxiety, dry mouth, sometimes-inappropriate giggles. But the side effects from an opioid prescription are much worse and are usually the reason why patients are so desperate to switch from pills to pot. Even on a good day, opioids can cause serious constipation, dizziness, nausea, and dopey confusion.

It can be difficult to recommend the right cannabis product and dose for pain, simply because all pain is different. A small dose—one inhalation or a small edible—is usually enough to knock out my menstrual cramps, but I need a bigger dose when my sciatic nerve pain flares up. One patient found that a cannabis-infused cream was strong enough to handle her arthritic hands, but she needed more marijuana to reduce the pain in her knees. Fibromyalgia patients, especially, seem to spend more time experimenting with several different forms of cannabis before they find the product that works for them, simply because everyone's fibromyalgia pain is different. Using a pain chart when you talk to your doctor or dispensary expert is a good place to start when describing your pain.

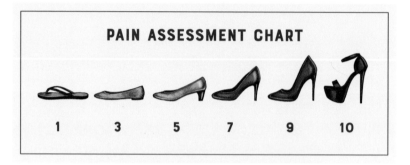

PAIN ASSESSMENT CHART

1   3   5   7   9   10

CANNABIS FOR A GOOD MOOD

Runners love to brag about their exercise-induced highs, but when they're huffing and puffing down the road, they're doing the exact same thing I'm doing. Except I'm sitting in a lawn chair and smoking a joint. They are improving their lung capacity. So am I. They are reducing stress and boosting their dopamine levels, just like I am. The running brain is flooded with endocannabinoids—naturally produced, medicinal compounds in the body that mimic compounds found in marijuana. I am flooding my brain with medicinal compounds from cannabis; plus I'm avoiding shin splints. And sweating.

Marijuana relieves the mood swings of menopause and can help treat postpartum depression. During my teenage years, I often asked my dad, in a very snotty tone, "What is *wrong* with Mom?" His answer always sounded so ominous. "The change."

Now that I've hit middle age with marijuana, I know how wrong he was. My mother had an obnoxious teenager, a husband who didn't understand her feelings, and no marijuana to help her body adjust to low estrogen levels, so her mood swings were awful.

Cannabis can be an excellent antidepressant and anti-anxiety medicine, but the dosage is critical. The euphoria and mood boost from cannabis can help lift stress, depression, and anxiety, without the side effects of prescription pills. But too much cannabis can increase anxiety and depression. Patients who show signs of lethargy and lack of motivation could be severely depressed, or they could be heavy marijuana users, because the symptoms are the same for both.

The Greeks taught us that moderation is the key to happiness, and this is especially true with marijuana. A small dose is relaxing and calming. A large dose is disorienting and anxiety inducing. In one study, anxiety increased with doses of 15 milligrams but was reduced in patients who took less than 10 milligrams. If you take a dose and feel uncomfortable, you've taken too much. It is not supposed to make you uncomfortable.

Some doctors think cannabis is a great alternative treatment for depression, but others disagree and point to marijuana dependence as a cause of depression, not a cure. Other doctors believe cannabis can help treat addiction. The research does not look good for cannabis use with schizophrenia or bipolar disorder.

Everybody is different, so talk with your doctor, honestly, about your specific medications, conditions, and cannabis use.

Right now, there is not a lot of medical research into cannabis and depression, and what we do have doesn't tell us much. There is a link between cannabis dependence and depression, but we don't know if cannabis causes the depression or if depressed patients choose to self-medicate with cannabis; we do know that the patients in the studies are self-medicating with illegal marijuana, not the more medicinal (and legal and better quality) marijuana available in dispensaries.

After twenty years of recreational and illegal marijuana use, I still had severe, chronic depression. Sometimes it was a low hum, just under the surface. I was able to function, but I hated everything and everyone. Sometimes I couldn't get off the couch for a week. It was not situational depression, because it followed me everywhere. I was depressed when I failed, but I was also depressed when I succeeded. But now, with the assistance of the right kind of medical marijuana, my depression has lifted. No antidepressant ever did that for me.

CANNABIS FOR ANTIAGING

A group of my mother's friends from college went to Colorado to celebrate their seventieth birthdays—on 4/20, the official marijuana holiday. They went to get high and have fun. They crashed at a granddaughter's house and Ubered to a dispensary to pick out brownies and candies and pre-rolled joints. Before they left, I went online and found a clean, upscale dispensary that was located just a few miles from the granddaughter's house.

"Ten-milligram edibles, no more. Do not eat another one for a full forty-five minutes." A couple of ladies wrote it down. Others darted their eyes at one another, and I knew I had found my troublemakers. "I mean it. Ten milligrams. If you ignore me, you will regret it."

I tried to get tough. "And no alcohol. None. That includes wine." More darting eyes. "You cannot get drunk and high at the same time. College kids have been trying and failing for decades. You are not stronger than they are. Weed only, ladies."

The ladies went to the mountains, got high, and had a grand time. Two of them bought a bottle of wine and vomited after drinking a glass while smoking a joint. All of them broke federal laws when they smuggled home topical creams in their suitcases.

And they aren't alone. Older people are trying marijuana, for medicine and for fun, in record numbers.

Some good news for those of us whose teen years are a distant memory: The research indicates, quite clearly, that cannabis is amazing for old brains—and not so great for young brains. Until your late twenties, the brain is still developing and getting smarter. Every day, neurons, nerves, and other important pieces of the brain make connections to build the brain into a fully developed muscle. When a teenager smokes weed, the brain abandons whatever connections it was going to make that day to get smarter and stronger. When teenagers become heavy, daily users of marijuana, they suffer later as adults. Less emotional development, less intelligence, less motivation—the typical stoner stereotype.

But if you are over forty now, your brain is fully developed, and the focus should be on protecting and preserving your brain so it works the way you want it to for as long as possible.

Cannabis is a strong antioxidant and reduces the plaque that builds up in the brain and causes dementia. It also reduces stress and inflammation, which are major factors in aging and decline. Cannabis is also a neuroprotective, which means it protects the brain against cognitive dysfunction like dementia and Alzheimer's. Older mice have shown memory and learning improvements with cannabis. While we are high, we lose short-term memory function, but once we come down, the cannabis has strengthened our short-term memory capabilities.

Cannabis can help prevent dementia from developing, and it can also help reduce the effects and symptoms of dementia like agitation and behavior issues. Some of the most exciting results of cannabis medicine have been with dementia patients, because the transformation is so quick and dramatic. One woman lived in a nursing home and was refusing to eat. She was so agitated the staff had to tie down her wrists so she wouldn't hurt herself. Her family brought some cannabis oil and gave her a few drops, and an hour later, her restraints were gone and she was smiling and happily eating orange slices.

As we get older, our skeleton grows weaker and more brittle, and our bones begin to hurt. Osteoporosis and arthritis slow us down, limit our range of motion, and cause debilitating pain. Cannabis can help strengthen our bones and joints as well as reduce pain in inflamed joints.

CANNABIS FOR WEIGHT LOSS

When I moved to Denver several years ago, two things happened. I started using medical marijuana for the first time, and I started losing weight. I didn't realize that the cannabis was the reason I was suddenly fitting into my college jeans; I just thought it was the altitude and new hiking hobby.

But then I moved to Illinois and didn't have access to medical cannabis anymore, just recreational. The weight came back with a vengeance. I blamed the lack of mountains and threw out the college jeans. My body started to hurt more, so I stopped exercising. I felt hungry all the time and needed more food to get through the day.

And then I fractured my spine. Exercise was no longer an option because I couldn't even stand up straight without pain. Because I felt so horrible, I ate whatever I wanted, whenever I wanted. My weight ballooned up to a new record high. I couldn't walk a mile without muscle spasms in my back and hips.

I wish I could say that I was self-motivated to get in shape and feel better, but I was not. I simply got my Illinois medical marijuana patient card and had access to medical cannabis again. I went to the dispensary, bought some flower, smoked it, and immediately felt better. The depression lifted. I finally felt ready to do the work to get in shape. That first walk, I came home and lay on my living room floor and cried over the shooting pain in my hips and back. For weeks, I went out every day and walked until I couldn't take the pain anymore. The first time I completed an easy, beginner yoga class, I was sore for a week. When I'm in shape, I can swim a mile in less than thirty minutes, so groaning and inching my way down the sidewalk for less than six blocks was humiliating. If I couldn't get the motivation to walk, I would smoke a joint and then force myself out the door.

After a month of grueling exercise, I lost ten pounds. I was still eating whatever I felt like eating, but the weight was coming off. I had read a few studies about the effects of marijuana on weight loss, so I decided to do an experiment on myself. I designed my own Cannabis Diet. Daily doses of cannabis, 1,200 calories a day (no food restrictions), a thirty-minute dog walk, and thirty minutes of yoga a day. Lots of water and sleep. I set my daily goals in my Fitbit, stocked up on cannabis oil, started counting calories, and let six months pass.

I lost fifty pounds.

I'm not gonna lie—it sucked. I was often hungry. There were cheat days. Sometimes I skipped going to a party because I knew that if I went, I would eat. I had dreams about carbs. But on most days I was able to stick to the calorie limit. I ate as much protein and fiber as I could, but some days (Halloween), I ate 1,200 calories of candy.

I hate diets. I hate counting calories, I hate Weight Watchers points. I make fun of vegans. I put butter on everything. If I am not allowed to eat a food, that is the only food I want. It only takes an hour of hunger for me to get angry about starving myself for the patriarchy and start posting Naomi Wolf quotes from *The Beauty Myth* on social media. Without cannabis, I cannot make it on 1,200 calories a day without losing my mind.

I get too hungry, too crabby, too mean. When I get enough cannabis, I'm more emotionally stable and balanced. Things don't bother me as much, and I can live with being hungry.

We all know about the marijuana-induced munchies. Marijuana is an appetite stimulant, and if you really want your dinner party guests to rave about your food, pass a joint around the table before the first course. Studies have shown that marijuana users eat several hundred more calories a day than non–marijuana users. They are enjoying their food, and they are eating more of it.

But cannabis users also have lower body mass indexes (BMIs) and smaller waistlines, despite their supersized meals. Even though I've always lived the hippie lifestyle, I'd never acquired that long and lean hippie body type. But when I started using CBD-rich cannabis, I lost weight. CBD (cannabidiol) is an appetite suppressant. THC (tetrahydrocannabinol) increases the desire to eat, but CBD reduces it. With a daily dose of cannabis oil in the morning, I am able to control what I put in my mouth and follow the diet and exercise plan. (I usually swipe 0.1 ml of oil on my gums. We'll get into why that's the best way to do it.) When I do want to eat past my calorie limit, I take a quick inhalation, and within minutes, I have enough willpower to resist food.

So far, the Cannabis Diet is a total success. I've lost weight, I can eat whatever I want as long as I stop at 1,200 calories, and everything tastes good. I can hike again, I can hold a plank for several minutes, and my back does not hurt.

The Olympic committee decided that athletes can use marijuana, just not on the day of their event. They don't consider marijuana a performance-enhancing drug. But many athletes, including professional players, think of cannabis as a performance recovery drug to heal their bodies after they train and compete. Out-of-shape couch potatoes feel like they're training at an Olympic level when they first get into shape, and they deserve cannabis for their efforts as much as gold medal winners.

CANNABIS FOR BEAUTY

A couple of years ago, I limped into my yoga studio, a lightning bolt of nerve pain shooting from my hip to my knee. I'd spent a week at my desk with a deadline, nonstop. My shoulders hunched into my ears and my humpback posture made the instructor wince. I rolled out my mat and spent ninety minutes stretching and releasing my breath and my muscles. Joints popped and cracked as I pushed through every range of motion. When I put my shoes back on, the nerve pain was gone; my back felt loose; and my head, neck, and shoulders were back in alignment. I smiled at the instructor on my way out.

"Oh, that looks much better," she said.

Hair and makeup can help, but Sephora can't give us the kind of beauty that comes from health, relaxation, and happiness. There's a reason we all use our vacation photos for social media profile pics—we always look so good on vacation. Necks and shoulders are relaxed, furrowed brows are smoothed out, and the only lines we see are smile lines. Getting high gets us to that same relaxed state without a plane ticket, and it shows on our faces.

Inhaling or eating cannabis makes a huge difference in our appearance. We can't hide stress and pain. They show up in our posture and our facial expressions. But cannabis reduces pain and stress and improves our mood, which stops the frowning. And when we start using cannabis, we start to sleep better, too.

Getting enough sleep is the single best thing we can do to improve our looks, and marijuana helps us get the sleep we need so in the morning we're well rested and ready to face a new day. Restorative night sleep and delightful daytime naps eliminate under-eye circles and bags, refresh skin, and give us the rest our body needs to function at full capacity.

My Fitbit tracks my sleep. It tells me how long I slept and how restless I was. I can easily see a pattern in the nightly graphs, a stark difference between the nights I take a bedtime dose of cannabis and nights when I don't. On cannabis nights I fall asleep faster, stay asleep longer, and spend less time tossing and turning.

But it doesn't end there. Serious skin conditions like eczema and psoriasis respond well to cannabis applied directly to the skin, and healthy skin looks younger and more beautiful with cannabis-infused skin products. The medicinal compounds in cannabis are anti-inflammatory, antibacterial, antifungal, and anti-aging. When we infuse cannabis into a cream or an oil, then use that cream as a daily moisturizer, we glow within days. Acne and redness disappear, dry patches are gone, and fine lines become finer. We can infuse cannabis into oils, lotions, and creams for our feet, legs, knees and elbows, backs, shoulders, necks, faces, and hands. These oils, lotions, and creams will relieve pain and inflammation and make us glow from head to toe.

After a long day in uncomfortable shoes, I soak my feet in a hot bath and then slather on a thick, rich cannabis-infused cream. I pull on socks and go to bed. In the morning, my feet are smooth, my ankles aren't swollen, and my toes don't hurt. I labeled it *Magic Trick* cream because I go to bed with forty-five-year-old feet, but I wake up with the feet of a twenty-five-year-old who is ready to work a double shift and then go dancing.

MOM AND WEED

In high school, my mom told me not to do drugs. In college, she got very upset when I used marijuana. Really upset. But recently, she told me the dog needed a dose of cannabis for his aching hips. People change. I don't care how conservative/religious/morally opposed to marijuana your mom is, if she is in pain, it will help her.

My mom's friends ask me for weed at twice the rate that my own friends ask, and only sometimes do they want it for fun. Usually, they want it because they heard that cannabis might reduce their pain. It's always pain that finally gets someone to try cannabis, whether that pain is a toothache, arthritis, or chemo.

Chances are good that if your mother qualifies for AARP, cannabis will improve her quality of life. Cannabis works its best magic on old brains and bodies. Many older people, however, are reluctant to change their minds about marijuana. They may consider it a kids' thing, or dangerous or potentially embarrassing—even if they tried it in their youth. It's not their fault: The anti-marijuana propaganda way back when was created with them in mind, so it takes them a bit longer to come around.

You don't want your mom to be in pain, but she might not be willing to try cannabis until her pain is more than she can bear. I began the marijuana conversation with my mother because my brother has seizures. For others, watching a loved one suffer through cancer is enough to change their minds about marijuana. But even if Mom has accepted that cannabis is medicine for others, she might not know that it can work for her, too. Sometimes a little nudge is all it takes.

How to Start the Conversation

STEP 1: COLLECT YOUR RESEARCH. Cannabis doesn't fix everything, but it helps with a lot of diseases and conditions. Start with your mom's major health issue—chronic pain, cancer, Parkinson's, seizures, dementia. Choose good sources, then take your evidence to Mom. Get her to read this book. My mom changed her mind when she saw a CNN documentary about CBD.

STEP 2: OVERCOME RESISTANCE. This requires patience and possibly several conversations to address her specific concerns. Show her success stories of other people, with her specific condition, who found relief. Remember to point out that it is impossible to overdose on marijuana, and it is actually one of the safest drugs she can try.

STEP 3: GET HER SIGNED UP FOR A PATIENT CARD. The process is different in every state, but worth the time and effort. Check the requirements for your state to see what kind of paperwork you need to gather and what kind of doctor you need to see.

STEP 4: START LOW, GO SLOW. If your mom has never smoked cigarettes, she won't want to start smoking now. Get her an edible, 5 to 10 milligrams of THC at most. (THC is tetrahydro-cannabinol—The High Creator. More on that later.) But if she was a cigarette smoker at any point in her life, she may feel comfortable smoking for her first time—and it's the fastest way to feel results. If she wants to vape, buy a cartridge and battery at the dispensary. If she's afraid to get high, stick with CBD-rich products. (More on this later!)

STEP 5: LEAVE HER ALONE. Give Mom her privacy. I know you want to see your mom get high, but she won't like it, so keep your chill.

STEP 6: GET HER TO DO IT AGAIN. If she experiences any adverse side effects, or doesn't feel anything at all, she might not want to try another dose. Encourage her to give cannabis another chance. Try a larger dose or a different strain. Try a muscle rub cream instead of an edible. Give the vape pen a shot.

STEP 7: DON'T GIVE HER MARIJUANA WITHOUT HER KNOWLEDGE. Everyone should give consent before they use a mind-altering substance, so do not attempt to prove how mild a strain is by giving her an edible without telling her it has cannabis in it. This is a bad plan. Keep it honest and respect her wishes.

Over the years, I have spoken to hundreds of people about medical marijuana. When women ask questions, sometimes they're asking for themselves, but at least half of them are talking about someone else. A lot of women are caretakers, and they're thinking about aging parents, a spouse in pain, or a child with cancer. Children are allowed medical marijuana, but two doctors are usually required to sign their recommendations. Later in the book we'll learn about which kinds of cannabis are appropriate for children. I've watched my own brother have daily seizures for forty-five years, so it is especially gratifying to talk to the mothers of children with seizures a few weeks after they get cannabis oil for their child. There is always crying during these conversations.

"She used to have fifty seizures a day. Now, she has one or two seizures a month! She's starting to talk!"

No matter if you're reading this book for yourself or for someone else, you will learn about how cannabis can help you and your loved ones. For many people, cannabis is a family affair.

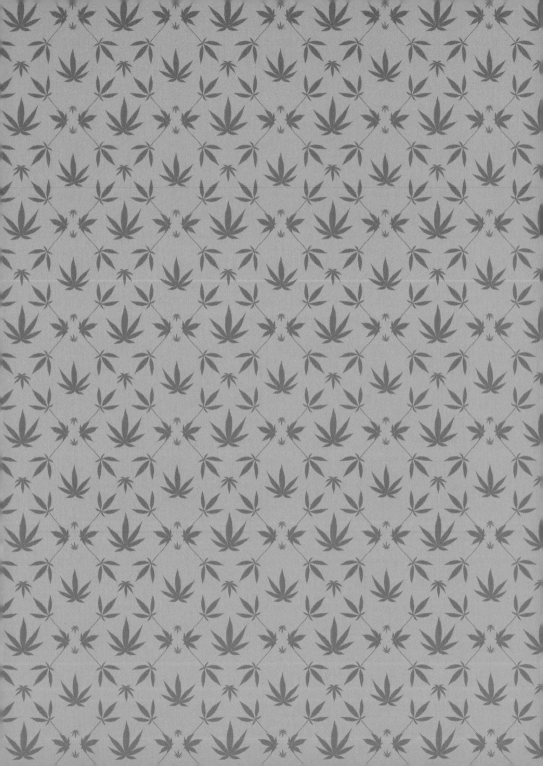

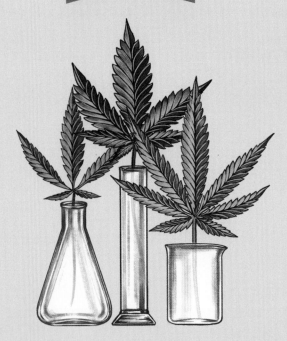

Part Two

HOW CANNABIS MAKES US HEALTHY AND HAPPY

People have used this magical flower for its medicinal healing properties for thousands of years, but it wasn't until the 1980s that scientists discovered and named some of the most important compounds in marijuana that make us feel healthier, happier, and high. After you finish this section of the book, you will know those compounds and what each of them does for you. You'll also learn a lot of the cannabis lingo that is used in dispensaries.

CANNABIS STRAINS

Golden Delicious, Gala, Fuji, McIntosh, Cortland, Jonagold, Red Delicious, Honeycrisp, Ginger Gold, Granny Smith, Jonathan, Arkansas Black. Do these names sound familiar? Apples come in dozens of varieties. They're all apples, but they're slightly different colors and flavors and shapes.

Cannabis is the same. Maui Wowie, Super Lemon Haze, Chocolope, Grape Ape, Girl Scout Cookies, Sour Diesel, Jack Herer, and Purple Trainwreck. Island Sweet Skunk, Strawberry Cough, and Matanuska Thunderfuck. It's all marijuana, but each strain gets us high in a slightly different way.

Cannabis strains are a bit like snowflakes—each one is unique, but very similar to the others. All strains are grown the same way, with the same plant structure and green flowers, but there are slight differences that you can see in the jars in the dispensary. Marijuana flowers from different strains are slightly different in color and size and density.

But the odor of a strain is the biggest difference. In some states you can open jars and smell the strains before you choose. Some smell sweet and citrusy while others smell like a park after a rainstorm. The odor of a strain can tell you what kind of high you'll get from it. Strains that smell earthy, like hops and floral, are relaxing. Strains that smell citrusy tend to be more energizing.

Cannabis sativa is the scientific name for this magical plant, but the flower itself has so many nicknames it's difficult to keep track. Cannabis, marijuana, pot, herb, weed, bud, MMJ, Mary Jane, flower, smoke. They all mean the exact same thing. In Aruba, a cabdriver made eye contact in the rearview mirror and, with such a charming smile, asked if I wanted ganja. It made me wish that was the only word we had for it.

Marijuana is an exotic Spanish word that was coined during Prohibition to associate cannabis with immigrants from Mexico. While the word has shed those racist roots, it's still suffering from poor publicity. Many adults prefer to use the word *cannabis.*

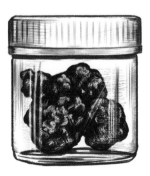

By the end of this section you will know which odors to sniff out to find the cannabis you want. You'll know how to read the test results and which kind of cannabis will work best for you.

We don't have specific strains for specific conditions—yet. My back pain disappears when I inhale Harlequin, but my friend doesn't feel any relief from her back pain with Harlequin. There is no strain specifically for epilepsy or arthritis. Your husband might love the antidepressant effects of Sour Diesel, while Sour Diesel just makes you feel paranoid and anxious.

To keep track of all these marijuana strains, dispensaries use a simple classification system. To understand this system, it's time to learn the difference between sativa and indica.

SATIVA IN THE MORNING, INDICA AT NIGHT

It is two in the morning and I am awake. I had a long day and I should be exhausted. But a couple of hours ago, I sampled a new strain, and now I'm focused and working. I'm in a great mood and I'm getting things done. I won't be sleeping anytime soon, and it's all because I sampled a sativa strain at midnight.

Sativa varieties of cannabis are as stimulating as a cup of coffee. They give us energy, lift our mood, inspire creativity, relieve depression, and give us the boost we need to have a good day. A sativa strain tends to be more of a cerebral, creative high. Your budtender will reach for a sativa if you say anything about medicating during the day. Recreational marijuana users like sativa-dominant strains for activities like socializing, exercise, and creative pursuits, but sativa strains can also increase anxiety if the dose is too high. Sour Diesel, Durban Poison, Super Lemon Haze, and Trainwreck are some of the most well-known sativa strains. One mnemonic for remembering sativa's effects is that *sateeva* rhymes with *acteeva*, which sounds like *activity*.

Indica varieties of cannabis, on the other hand, have the opposite effect. They are relaxing, relieve stress, and encourage sleep. An indica high is described as a "body high." Tension melts from the muscles, and it relaxes motivation. If you tell a budtender you want to sleep at night, they will immediately grab an indica off the shelf and start talking about "couch-lock"—the sensation of becoming so relaxed that getting off the couch is a monumental accomplishment. These sleepy-time strains are perfect for anxiety, insomnia, and pain. When I'm going for a massage or climbing into a bathtub, I choose indica strains to encourage relaxation. Peaceful, restorative sleep is the best medicine, and indica strains are the ones that get us there. Strains like Blueberry, Kosher Kush, and Granddaddy Purps are great indicas for sleep. You can remember what an indica is for by thinking *indica-indigo-nighttime*.

Hybrids are a mix of indica and sativa, so they're a little bit relaxing and also a little bit stimulating. Some hybrids are more one or the other; indica dominant means that strain is more relaxing than invigorating. If something is labeled *sativa dominant* it means that strain isn't going to help you nap. Most strains that are available on the legal market are hybrids, and purely indica or sativa strains are rare.

People prefer indica or sativa for particular conditions or individual taste, but most people use both, depending on the type of high they're looking for and what they want to do while they're high. When I go to a Vinyasa class to flow and burn off some energy, I reach for a sativa. When I go to a restorative yoga class to relax and relieve stress, I inhale an indica. At the dispensary, I'll buy a container of a sativa strain and another container of an indica strain so I have both at home. When I want a hybrid, I mix a little from each jar.

Unless I have Blue Dream, and then I just smoke that. If the *New York Times* had a bestseller list for marijuana strains, Blue Dream would have been comfortably ensconced in the top five since at least 2013. Blue Dream smells like lavender and is a slightly milder high than other strains. Getting high with Blue Dream makes you feel relaxed and creative and puts you in a good mood. The strain gets its name from its parents— Blueberry and Haze. When a mommy plant and a daddy plant love each other very much, the male plant releases pollen and the female plant uses the pollen to grow seeds. Those seeds are planted, and the resultant baby plant is a mixture, a hybrid, of the two strains used to create it. Blueberry is an indica that relieves pain and relaxes the body, while Haze is a creative sativa. Mixing the two creates the perfect hybrid that manages to please just about everyone.

In the dispensary, cannabis flowers are sorted into three simple categories: sativa, indica, or hybrid. Most dispensaries have at least four to five strains available in each category, and some have over a dozen. I love Granddaddy Purps for my regular indica. But sometimes when I stop by the dispensary, they

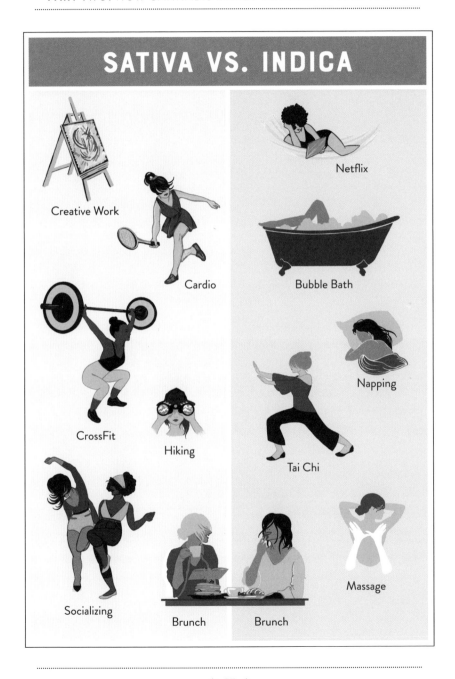

don't have any Granddaddy Purps that day, so I have to get a different indica.

The indica/sativa/hybrid classification system basically works, but it isn't the most accurate way to do it. Before lab testing became a standard practice in the marijuana industry, no one knew what made an indica an indica or a sativa a sativa. When we smoked a new marijuana strain and fell asleep, it was an indica. If we smoked a new strain and wrote a song, it was a sativa.

Now consumers know that cannabinoids and terpenes are the medicinal compounds in cannabis (more detail on these compounds to come). They get us high, make us relaxed, and give us the munchies. Knowing this, we can look to the lab testing results instead of our noses to find the best strain for us.

THE ENDOCANNABINOID SYSTEM

From the dawn of time until 1937, cannabis had been used to improve health, wellness, and beauty. Queen Victoria used a marijuana tincture to relieve her menstrual cramps. It's been said that JFK sparked up in the White House to cope with pain. Marijuana has been found in ancient tombs. Until Prohibition, pharmacies were well stocked with marijuana tinctures and creams, and apothecaries created custom-made marijuana medicine.

Our bodies like cannabis so much, we have an entire system to use it. The endocannabinoid system of our bodies works like a lock and key. The locks are receptors that are located in our brains, central nervous systems, and throughout the body. They are called CB1 and CB2 receptors. Cannabis is the key. When we consume marijuana, the medicinal compounds move through the bloodstream until they find and lock into those CB1 and CB2 receptors in our bodies, and we get high, our pain disappears, and we feel better.

The endocannabinoid system helps to maintain homeostasis throughout the entire body, a stable balance in which every system is working efficiently. Disease is a result of an imbalance of homeostasis—when something in the body is off kilter. The endocannabinoid system recognizes the imbalance and works to help correct it. Studies have shown that when conditions like pain, anxiety, arthritis, and MS develop in the body, the endocannabinoid system responds by creating more receptors and endocannabinoids to make us feel better and reduce pain. One theory floating around the cannabis research community is that many conditions and diseases are simply the result of a cannabinoid deficiency in the body, and that maintaining a strong endocannabinoid system is just as important as maintaining a good immune system.

Cannabis plants aren't the only things that make feel-good compounds. The human body itself is basically a plant that produces many natural compounds, one of which is anandamide (pronounced ah-NAN-dah-mide, and Sanskrit for *inner bliss*). It works just like compounds from the cannabis plant. Anandamide compounds regulate mood, sleep, pain, appetite, and other functions, just like cannabis. Breast milk contains anandamide compounds that assist newborns with suckling, while other endocannabinoids assist in the regulation of inflammation, immune function, and thermoregulation.

THC: THE QUEEN BEE CBD: THE VALEDICTORIAN

There are literally hundreds of medicinally beneficial compounds in marijuana, but two of them do most of the work: THC and CBD. They are the two main cannabinoids in cannabis. As I said, cannabinoids are the keys—the chemical compounds that lock into receptors in your body and activate your endocannabinoid system.

THC is the queen bee of her high school because she decides how long the party lasts and which days we wear pink. THC (it stands for *tetrahydrocannabinol*, but it's easier to remember it as The High Creator) is the only compound in cannabis that is psychoactive, so it is the only compound that gets us high. The psychoactive effect happens when dopamine floods the brain and we feel pleasure, joy, euphoria. We relax, food tastes better, and everything is funny.

We used to think that CBD (cannabidiol) was just another wannabe cannabinoid trailing behind the glamorous THC. But in recent years, CBD has become the valedictorian of her class—the brightest star with the most potential. CBD initially gained recognition because of its ability to reduce seizures, but that's just the beginning of what CBD can do. CBD reduces inflammation and pain, arthritis, muscle spasms, and epilepsy, and also fights cancer cells. CBD is a bone stimulant and helps reduce blood sugar levels, which controls and prevents diabetes.

THC and CBD have many of the same benefits. They are both analgesic, antioxidant, and anti-inflammatory. They are both powerful antidepressants and reduce anxiety. They are antibacterial, which means they can reduce gum disease, heart disease, and intestinal disease. THC and CBD decrease nausea and are powerful antispasmodics that control neurological excitability and reduce seizures, muscle spasms, and tremors. THC and CBD are both neuroprotective and reduce nervous system degeneration, and they slow the production of amyloid plaque that leads to dementia.

The difference is that THC makes us high, but CBD does not. CBD does not give us the giggles or the munchies like THC. While THC is out partying, CBD is at home getting her homework done. But when they work together, when THC is consumed with CBD, they bring out the best in each other. Adding CBD to THC enhances and extends the high, so we feel better for longer. CBD smooths out the negative side effects of THC, like anxiety.

CBD-rich cannabis is like heirloom vegetables. Wild cannabis plants have a balanced amount of THC and CBD. But starting in the eighties, when illegal marijuana cultivators brought their plants indoors to protect them from law enforcement detection, growers began cultivating strains with more THC and less CBD. For decades, marijuana cultivators have selected the plant that got them higher than the other plants and bred them with other "dude, we got so high from that one" plants. Eventually, this genetic selection resulted in highly potent marijuana with very little CBD.

Now, because of the new popularity of CBD, cannabis breeders and growers are cultivating CBD-rich plants, so we're slowly headed back to the genetics of cannabis plants that grew wild and were harvested for medicines before 1937.

EFFECTS OF THC	EFFECTS OF CBD
High	Antidepressant
Sleep	Antianxiety
Pain relief	Pain relief
Appetite stimulant	Appetite suppressant
Stress relief	Stress relief
Reduces tremors and seizures	Reduces tremors and seizures
Antiaging	Antiaging

Potency

The most important characteristic of a strain is the potency—how much THC and CBD are in that particular strain. To get high, we eat or smoke the flowers of a female marijuana plant, and the amount of THC determines how high we get. Potency is the amount of a drug needed for a certain effect and intensity.

A lower potency drug produces a milder effect, while a higher potency medicine produces the desired effect at a lower dose.

Cannabis flower potency is expressed in percentages and can be anywhere from 1 to 30 percent THC, which means that THC is 1 to 30 percent of the total weight of the flower. When marijuana is 5 percent THC, it means 50 of the 1,000 milligrams in a gram of flower are THC. Twenty percent potency means that each gram of flower contains 200 milligrams of THC. If we inhale one hit of 20 percent THC marijuana, we get very high quickly. If we inhale one hit of 5 percent THC marijuana, we get a little bit high.

In the sixties, marijuana potency was about 2 to 8 percent THC. One joint—a single gram of cannabis—was enough to get three people mildly high. By the nineties, marijuana potency was creeping up to 10 to 15 percent THC, so those three people would get really high with a gram-sized joint. Today, marijuana potency in dispensaries is anywhere from 15 to 30 percent THC. One 25 percent THC joint will get our little gang very, very high. For some people, it's too high.

This increasing potency isn't a bad thing—it just means we don't have to inhale or eat as much marijuana to get the same effect. If you smoked marijuana in college, but college was more than a few years ago, don't think you can inhale as much as you did back in the day.

CBD potency is measured the same way, by percentage. Some strains have just a little bit of CBD—1 to 5 percent. Some strains have balanced, equal amounts of THC and CBD, 5 to 10 percent of each, and some strains are just a little bit THC and a lot CBD.

LEVELS OF HIGH
VERY HIGH = high THC + low CBD
MILD HIGH = even balance of THC + CBD
NOT HIGH = low THC + high CBD

BY THE NUMBERS
VERY HIGH: 10–30% THC (*a lot*) + 0–2% CBD
(*not a lot*)
MILD HIGH: 5–15% THC + 5–15% CBD
(*even amount for both*)
NOT HIGH: 1–5% THC (*not a lot*) + 5–30% CBD (*a lot*)

HIGH-THC, LOW-CBD cannabis strains are the most popular strains because they are the most fun. THC gets us high, but it can also cause anxiety if we take too much. Many people buy marijuana with the most THC because they think they will get higher. But the truth is, we can only get so high. The endocannabinoid system only has so many receptors and can only absorb so many milligrams of THC at once. If we consume more than this, the THC is redirected and stored in our fat cells.

LOW-THC, HIGH-CBD cannabis strains make us feel better without getting us high. CBD strains are used to make cannabis medicine for children and anyone supervising children or operating heavy machinery. I reach for a CBD strain when I'm doing anything that requires a sober, clear mind.

1:1 THC/CBD (one-to-one) cannabis strains are the most medicinally beneficial strains for almost everyone. They have a mild high and a lot of pain relief. The first time I inhaled a 1:1 strain, I felt pretty good. Just a little high, and my shoulders instantly dropped and relaxed. With the second inhalation, the blanket of depression lifted from my shoulders.

Back then, Harlequin was one of the only 1:1 strains available in dispensaries. These days, there are more 1:1 strains to choose from.

Sharon got her medical card because her oncologist and her kids told her that marijuana would make her feel better, but she was not convinced. Sharon was a retired high school math teacher, and after supervising the D.A.R.E. program for so many years, Sharon did not believe that marijuana could possibly be medicine. She was as suspicious about medical marijuana as she was about her students' missing homework, but the chemo was more painful than she expected, so she reluctantly agreed to at least give marijuana a try.

"I don't want to get high. I don't drink alcohol, because I don't like how it makes me feel," Sharon said. "I like to feel in control."

"You don't have to get high, and you don't have to smoke it," I said, as I gathered up a selection of CBD edibles and answered her next objection before she said it.

"And I don't want candy either," she said. "It's just not right to make marijuana appealing to children."

I nodded my head and put back the gummy candy. I showed her a small bottle of liquid tincture and pulled out a magnifying glass so she could see the label. "THC is the only thing that gets us high, so you just have to make sure that you take less than five milligrams of THC at a time," I said. I showed her how to squeeze the dropper top on the tincture for a single dose. Each dose had 1 milligram of THC and 20 milligrams of CBD. Sharon bought the tincture, tucked it into her purse, and slipped out of the dispensary like a ninja, afraid someone she knew might see her.

When Sharon came back the second time, she was a little more comfortable with everything. She wasn't hiding behind sunglasses, at least. But the chemo was starting to wear her down, and she looked pale.

"I feel better during the day," she said, when I asked her how she was feeling. "But I'm not sleeping well at all, and the nausea is worse than they said it would be."

"CBD is wonderful and miraculous, but it is not effective for insomnia or nausea. That's what THC is for," I said. She opened her mouth to object. "But if you take it before you go to bed, you'll sleep through the high." I pulled out a package of mints and showed Sharon the label. "Five milligrams of THC per mint," I said. "Eat one, just one, an hour or two before you go to bed. And keep taking the tincture in the morning."

"I slept through the night!" Sharon called the dispensary at ten a.m. the next morning. "I feel great! I got a little dizzy when I got into bed, but I fell asleep right away and when I woke up I felt like I was on vacation."

Sharon stuck to her tincture and mint schedule through her chemo. When her scans came back clear, she celebrated and continued to take marijuana because it made her feel better. A few months after she celebrated her scans, she brought a friend to the dispensary. "This is Deb, we used to teach together. She's stage 1, just like I was. She's here to get her tincture and mints." Sharon smiled and squeezed Deb's hand. "Don't be nervous," she said. "You'll barely feel the marijuana, but you'll feel so much better."

In the dispensary, the potency of the various flowers for sale is listed in a menu or displayed next to the flower under a glass case. Some states require lab testing for potency, and some do not. If your state does, the potency of the flower is listed on the package label.

THC and CBD are the main cannabinoids in cannabis, but others, listed on the following pages, are just as beneficial to our health and wellness. Some cannabis strains have a full range of cannabinoids, while others only have THC. In the dispensary, lab testing results show the exact potency of each cannabinoid. Some edibles, tinctures, and oils are focused on these less noticed cannabinoids. Keep this list handy and you'll be able to request more customized strains—or at least know what you're getting.

Minor Cannabinoids

- **CBC** (cannabichromene)—CBC inhibits cancer cell growth; promotes bone growth; and reduces inflammation, pain, and depression. CBC is ten times more powerful than CBD at reducing anxiety and stress and is the third most plentiful cannabinoid in marijuana. CBC boosts the effectiveness of other cannabinoids, which means it increases the psychoactive effect from THC.

- **CBG** (cannabigerol)—CBG not only inhibits the growth of cancer cells, but it also relieves pain from glaucoma, aids sleep, promotes bone growth, and slows bacterial growth. CBG is an antidepressant, increasing serotonin levels in the brain and preventing the uptake of amino acids that regulate mood. The exciting thing about CBG is that it is the only cannabinoid that stimulates the growth of new brain cells.

- **CBN** (cannabinol)—CBN is known for being the Ambien of cannabinoids, but it's more than just a sedative. CBN also stimulates the appetite, is an effective pain reliever, and can delay amyotrophic lateral sclerosis (ALS) symptoms. CBN prefers the CB2 receptor in the endocannabinoid system, so it has a greater effect on the immune system than it does on the central nervous system.

- **THCV** (tetrahydrocannabivarin)—THCV is going to become one of the most talked-about cannabinoids. Diet books will be written about it. THCV decreases body fat and reduces appetite and is currently being researched as a treatment for metabolic disorders, including diabetes. Not just for weight control, THCV is also an analgesic, anti-inflammatory, and anticonvulsant, and is neuroprotective, like THC and CBD. It also increases feelings of euphoria.

- **THCA** (tetrahydrocannabinolic acid)—Nonpsychoactive, THCA is the raw, acid form of THC. THCA reduces inflammation, muscle spasms, and the growth of tumors. Juicing and topicals are the most popular ways to consume the raw, acid forms of marijuana.

- **CBDA** (cannabidiolic acid)—Like THCA, CBDA is a powerful anti-inflammatory, inhibits cancer cell and bacterial growth, and reduces nausea and vomiting.

DO I SMELL POT? THE MAGIC AND SCIENCE OF TERPENES

My mom visited Denver for my birthday. After dinner downtown, we walked to the car. "I smell a skunk," she said. My mother has never smelled a skunk. She thinks camping is when the door to the hotel room opens directly to the outdoors.

"No, you don't," I said, as someone walked past us, a trail of smoke behind them. "You smell marijuana." A few months later, we were walking through the botanical gardens in Saint Louis.

"I smell marijuana." My mom sniffed the air.

"I think that might actually be a skunk," I said.

Cannabinoids do the heavy lifting, but terpenes (pronounced TER-pen-eez, and the singular is TER-pen-ee) are a vital part of marijuana medicine and the compound that gives marijuana its distinctive odor. Our bodies love cannabinoids, but we love terpenes even more. Even if you have never tried cannabis, you have consumed terpenes in fruit, spices, beer, and perfumes. The glands that produce cannabinoids also produce aromatic organic hydrocarbons that smell like pine, hops, mint, and berries. Take a stroll down the essential oil aisle at Whole Foods to smell different terpenes.

Terpenes offer an array of medicinal benefits.

Each strain of cannabis has its own particular terpene profile—a combination of dozens of terpenes that give each strain a distinctive odor. Most strains have some myrcene and pinene in them, but some might have just a bit of each while others have a high amount of one or the other. Lots of pinene gives us an alert, focused high while myrcene is sedating, so a jar of cannabis that smells like a pine forest will have a much different effect than a jar of cannabis that smells like cloves. A variety of marijuana strains will provide a well-rounded diet of terpenes. Almost all terpenes are anti-inflammatory, antifungal, antibacterial, and powerful antioxidants, in addition to the unique medicinal benefits they each have.

When the lab tests for cannabinoid potency, they also test to see how much of each terpene is in the cannabis. Most cannabis strains have an abundance of one or two terpenes, a medium amount of two to three terpenes, and a small amount of three to four terpenes. If you are looking for one particular terpene, ask your budtender if any strain has a high amount of it. If she doesn't know, and she doesn't have potency testing for terpenes, go by smell.

Even without test results, your nose will tell you which terpenes are in the flower. A lovely citrus fragrance signals that you're smelling limonene and that the strain is a sativa; if you notice a hoppy smell that reminds you of beer, then you're smelling myrcene, which indicates the strain is an indica. Caryophyllene gives off a distinct black pepper smell, which makes it easy to find among the jars in the dispensary. My favorite diet advice is to eat whatever you want because your body is telling you what you need. When it comes to marijuana, your nose will tell you what you need. Choose strains that smell good to you.

MYRCENE is in almost every strain and is also found in mango, lemongrass, bay leaves, eucalyptus, thyme, and hops. It smells like cloves, with an herbal, musky odor that contributes to the typical skunk smell of marijuana. Myrcene is a sedative and muscle relaxant, so cannabis with high myrcene levels creates a relaxing, sleepy effect while low myrcene levels have a more energetic, creative effect. Terpenes that have a sedative effect are also usually anticonvulsant, which reduces seizures and overactive brain activity. Myrcene also works to reduce tumors and is a strong soldier in the fight against cancer. It is anti-inflammatory, antiseptic, antibacterial, and antifungal.

The amount of myrcene is the main difference between an indica or a sativa strain. High levels of myrcene create a more relaxing indica high while low levels of myrcene result in more energizing highs, like sativa strains.

Try eating mango when using cannabis. Mango is loaded with myrcene, which lowers the blood-brain barrier resistance and allows cannabinoids and terpenes to quickly and easily cross the barrier, which speeds up the time it takes to get high and increases the high.

PINENE is in most cannabis strains and smells like pine, conifer, and fir, with a hint of sage. Pinene is in pine needles, rosemary, basil, parsley, and dill and is known for mental alertness, memory retention, and counteracting negative THC effects like anxiety. Many people use marijuana to treat attention deficit disorder (ADD), and pinene is the reason why. It helps us focus.

Pinene is an analgesic, anti-inflammatory, antioxidant, antiproliferative, and a bronchodilator, which increases airflow to the lungs and helps relieve asthma. Pinene may be one of the reasons why smoking marijuana has not been proven to cause harm to the lungs. It is usually abundant in sativa strains.

LIMONENE is the most important terpene for depression and anxiety and smells like its namesake—lemons. Limonene is in fruit rinds, rosemary, juniper, peppermint, and pine needle oils. When a strain is high in limonene, it produces a lift in mood and relieves depression, anxiety, and stress. It also dissolves gallstones and may treat gastrointestinal complications, acid reflux, and heartburn. Limonene increases blood flow from the heart, fights cancer, and stimulates the immune system.

Limonene is wonderful in skin treatments because it works synergistically to assist the absorption of other terpenes through the skin and suppresses the growth of fungi and bacteria, making it a powerful antifungal. Sativa strains are usually higher in limonene.

CARYOPHYLLENE gives black pepper a spicy kick and is also found in cloves, hops, cotton, rosemary, and basil. Caryophyllene is gastroprotective and helps relieve ulcers, autoimmune disorders, and gastrointestinal complications. This spicy terpene has anticancer properties, is a powerful muscle relaxant, and regulates lipids, which may mitigate or delay the onset of diabetes. Caryophyllene is the only terpene that interacts with the endocannabinoid system, as it binds to the CB2 receptors, making it both a terpene and a cannabinoid, like a mutant superhero. Indica strains tend to have more caryophyllene.

LINALOOL is the lavender of marijuana and a sedative that produces calming effects that relieve anxiety and depression and reduce seizures. Linalool strengthens the immune system, reduces lung inflammation, and is useful in treating Alzheimer's and other forms of dementia. Linalool is in birch trees, tropical plants, laurels, cinnamon, and rosewood. Read the ingredients on the shampoo bottles in your bathroom, and you'll find linalool listed as linalyl alcohol, linaloyl oxide, and alloocimenol. Linalool is a terpene that gives indica strains their sleepy, relaxing effects.

THE ENTOURAGE EFFECT: BRINGING IT ALL TOGETHER

Mother Nature is a mad scientist with cannabis strains. Each variety, or strain, of cannabis has cannabinoids and terpenes. What makes them different from one another is the amount of each cannabinoid and terpene in each strain. Some have lots of THC, no CBD, and a little CBN, with lots of myrcene and caryophyllene and just a bit of humulene. Others have very little THC, lots of CBD, a little CBG and CBC, sprinkled with pinene, limonene, and terpinolene.

When various cannabinoids and terpenes are combined into a specific cannabis strain, they work together to boost the effectiveness of each medicinal compound. When several analgesic cannabinoids and terpenes are abundant in a strain, it makes each compound stronger, so the overall effect is more potent. CBD by itself is a lovely pain reliever, but CBD and myrcene together are much more powerful.

A strain with 15 percent THC is no different than the 15 percent THC in another strain. But CBN is a strong sedative, so 15 percent THC and 2 percent CBN will feel more relaxing than THC alone. Marijuana with 15 percent THC and a healthy amount of pinene and limonene will result in an uplifting, energetic high and smoke that smells citrusy and piney. Fifteen percent THC with myrcene smells more hoppy and relaxes us right into sleep.

If individual cannabinoids or terpenes are isolated from other cannabinoids and terpenes, that compound will be less effective than medicine with a full range of cannabinoids and terpenes. THC or CBD only, without any terpenes, is less powerful than medicine with a full range of cannabinoids and terpenes. Ten milligrams of THC will provide a certain amount of pain relief, but if CBC and myrcene are included, those same 10 milligrams will provide even more pain relief that lasts longer. Hemp products that contain only CBD are not as effective as CBD-rich marijuana products that also have limonene and pinene.

This is why hemp products aren't as effective as marijuana products. Hemp has only small amounts of CBD and no THC or terpenes, which means we need a lot more hemp-based CBD to equal the same effects of marijuana CBD.

Someday, the combined efforts of medical and botanical research will create cannabis strains with the exact ratios of cannabinoids and terpenes that work for specific conditions and diseases, but that is still several years in the future. Until then, we each have to experiment with marijuana until we find cannabis strains and products that are most effective for us.

HEMP VS. CANNABIS

Margie lives in Illinois, and a few years ago, as her fibromyalgia and arthritis got steadily worse, she began taking an extra pain pill every day. She saw the slippery slope she was on and got worried that things were going to get worse. Margie's sister Kate had retired to Arizona and gotten herself a medical marijuana card to soothe her Parkinson's tremors. Kate was taking a daily dose of THC/CBD oil that relaxed her tremors and improved her mood. On the phone one day, Margie complained about the winter cold and the pain in her hands. Since Margie was still waiting for her medical marijuana card and couldn't purchase the same oil Kate was using, Kate told her to go to a health-food store and buy legal CBD oil, which has no THC.

At the health-food store, Margie found a small bottle by the register with CBD on it. It was labeled *hemp oil*. She picked it up and studied the label. It didn't say how much CBD was in the bottle or how much to take. It cost eighty dollars, but Margie was desperate. She bought it and took it home. She squeezed a dropper of oil into her mouth and waited an hour. Nothing happened. Her pain was still bad. She took another dose. Nothing.

A few weeks later, Margie went to Arizona to escape the midwestern winter cold and visit Kate. Margie told Kate about how the hemp oil didn't work, and so they decided to trade medicines to see if it was them or the oil. Margie took a dropper of oil from Kate's bottle of cannabis medicine, while Kate took a dropper of Margie's hemp oil medicine.

Two hours later, the cannabis oil had completely knocked out Margie's pain, but the hemp oil didn't help Kate at all. The sisters had to take almost the entire bottle of hemp oil to feel any sort of relief, while the cannabis oil worked effectively with a small dose.

Cannabis plants produce a lot more CBD. Hemp oil isn't effective because it just isn't potent enough. When hemp plants are processed and concentrated into oil, that oil just doesn't have anywhere near as many milligrams of CBD as cannabis oil. A bottle of cannabis tincture can have 500 to 1,000 milligrams of CBD while the same amount of hemp oil might have just 50 to 100 milligrams of CBD.

Cannabis plants produce a lot more CBD than hemp plants do.

The second reason that hemp isn't as effective as cannabis is because hemp doesn't have other cannabinoids like THC, CBN, CBC, and CBG, and hemp doesn't have terpenes like myrcene, pinene, and limonene. CBD works so much more effectively with just a little bit of THC. Remember the entourage effect—cannabis medicine is more potent and effective when it contains a full range of cannabinoids and terpenes, not just one isolated compound like CBD.

The cultivation of hemp plants and the processing of hemp oil are not regulated in the United States. Most CBD hemp oil is imported from other countries. No one knows what is in the hemp oil, because no one knows where it was grown or how it was made. Hemp oil is not tested for contaminants like mold and pesticides. Toxic pesticides are sprayed on the hemp plants and concentrated into the oil, which means that bottle from the health-food store may contain more pesticides than CBD.

Even though cannabis CBD is much better than hemp CBD, people who live in states without medical marijuana don't have a choice. Legal cannabis is highly regulated by the states and banned by the federal government, so it takes years of effort by activists to get medical marijuana laws in place, and then it takes another few years and millions of dollars to build the cultivations, processing centers, and dispensaries to get high-quality, highly effective cannabis medicine into the hands of patients.

Hemp CBD does not face these regulatory hurdles. Hemp is a gray area, not quite cannabis yet not quite legal. Proponents of hemp oil argue that the "illegal" compound in cannabis is THC, so if there is no THC, it is legal.

When someone is desperate, someone else is always ready to take advantage of that desperation. CBD-hemp-oil sales started online, but soon CBD hemp was available in independent health-food and vape stores. Then, CBD-hemp salesmen came calling. A few major cities have entire retail stores dedicated to CBD-hemp products, like dispensaries without the rules or effective medicine.

I'm not telling you not to take CBD hemp, but I won't advise it either. Hemp is great, and farmers should be allowed to grow it for paper and hippie clothes and vegan shoes, but it's not something we want to consume as medicine, especially when we have something so much better: cannabis.

Back in Illinois, Margie thought about getting cannabis oil in the mail from her sister, but neither one of them wanted to break the law, so Margie settled for CBD hemp until she was able to get her medical marijuana card last year. Once she was able to shop in a dispensary for cannabis oil with a full range of cannabinoids and terpenes, Margie never went back to hemp.

WHAT DO I TAKE
FOR . . . ?

I walked into the dispensary one day and found five women sitting in the lobby and having a heated argument. They all had notebooks in their laps and pens in their hands, and their voices were getting louder as all of them talked at one another and no one listened. I ducked into the employee break room to avoid getting sucked into the discussion before clocking in for the day.

"What is happening out there?" I asked a coworker as I shed my coat and snow boots.

"The patient review board finally sampled the suppositories," he said. "And all hell broke loose. You better talk to them."

There's a certain kind of shopper, and every retail employee has met her. She is high maintenance and demanding. As a stereotype, she is middle aged, type A, and ready to ask for the manager. She will make your life miserable if you don't please her, but she is actually a wonderful resource if you use her powers for good.

At the dispensary, we gathered all these opinionated ladies into a group and gave them new products to test. If they liked them, we stocked them in the store. If they didn't, we didn't. The group sampled new strains of flower, new vape pen cartridges, and new lotions. The ladies had lots of opinions on the packaging, the price, and the high, and they were always right. If they liked something, it sold like crazy. If they didn't like a product, no one else bought it either.

One lady was a cancer survivor, and another was just starting chemo. We had a Crohn's patient, a trauma survivor with PTSD, and a woman with ALS. The fibromyalgia patient didn't always show up to meetings, but would email her opinions to the group. None of them had tried cannabis before getting their patient card, so everything was new to them. At the first meeting, they had an idea.

None of them had tried cannabis before.

"We should create a list of strains and products that work for each of our conditions," said the cancer patient as they settled into their chairs. "And put it on the internet so everyone can see it." The rest of the group murmured their approval.

"Unfortunately, it doesn't quite work that way," I said. "Let's take an example. How many of you have tried Girl Scout Cookies?" More than half of the group raised their hand. "Did it work for you?" Most of the hands stayed up. "I hated it," I said. "It made me feel foggy and dumb, but not relaxed. It didn't help my pain, and it didn't make me feel better." Another woman nodded her head—it hadn't helped her either.

"I love it," said the woman with ALS. "It's the only thing that helps my muscle spasms."

"Maybe Girl Scout Cookies is the ALS strain," said another, and the group got excited. They decided to set up a corkboard in the lobby so other patients could tell them which strain worked for them, and what disease or condition they took it for.

Chaos ensued.

None of the other ALS patients liked Girl Scout Cookies, but one arthritis patient loved it, and a single cancer patient claimed it boosted her appetite. Over the course of a month, patients filled the corkboard with notes and the product-review group tried to keep them neat and organized. Dozens of cancer patients recommended their favorite products for chemo days, and none of them recommended the same thing. Ten glaucoma patients recommended ten different strains.

Debbie, the alpha of the group, stood in front of the corkboard and muttered to herself, "This isn't working." I came back a few minutes later and she had a new plan. "By symptom," she said. "We'll see what everyone uses for insomnia, for nausea, whatever."

A month later, the board was covered in notecards with no discernible way to organize the information. "No one can agree on a good strain for nausea," Debbie said. "The insomnia list is just a list of all the indica strains in the store, and the anxiety list is giving me anxiety."

Eventually, the group gave up on the corkboard. They still reviewed and evaluated new strains and products, and noted the effects they felt with each, but they knew that just because a particular strain made them feel sleepy and happy didn't mean it would make everyone feel sleepy and happy. Cannabis medicine is not exact or precise. There is not one strain that works for everyone with the same condition or disease. When you find what works for you, great. Try new things, sample edibles and strains that your friends like, but make sure to listen to your own body first.

TOLERANCE

"Don't take anything personally today. I have horrible cramps and I feel mean," I said to my friend Susan as we loaded the car for a day of hiking with our dogs.

"Me too," she said. "I brought gummies for that exact reason." She pulled a package from her purse and handed it to me. I checked the label—10 milligrams of THC in each candy.

"Those won't touch it," I said and handed them back. I pulled a syringe of oil from my own purse and squirted a dab of oil, the size of a grain of rice, onto my finger and then rubbed the oil into my gums. The dab of oil contained 20 milligrams of THC and 20 milligrams of CBD, the dose I needed to knock out menstrual cramps, and four times the number of milligrams that worked for Susan's cramps.

"What's that? Let me try it," Susan said.

"It's CO_2 oil. I need more than ten milligrams of THC, and I need CBD to knock out the cramps, and I don't want to eat all your gummies." I squeezed out a small dose for Susan, and she rubbed it into her gums.

We drove to the hiking trail and started walking. Susan didn't make it very far before she sat down on a rock. "Too high," she said and pulled out her water bottle. I am tall, big boned, and chubby, and I've been taking very high doses of THC for quite some time. Susan is petite and thin and just recently started using cannabis. She doesn't need nearly as much THC as I do, and that is fine. Everybody is different, so what works for you may not work for someone else.

Tolerance is how much of a drug it takes to feel effects and is partly dependent on the size of your body and partly dependent on your endocannabinoid system. Some people have more cannabinoid receptors than others, which means more THC can lock into the body at a time, so those people don't need as much marijuana to get high.

Smaller bodies with less body fat usually do better with smaller doses. Older bodies usually feel more comfortable with a smaller dose than younger bodies. Some people feel too high with 10 milligrams of THC, while others need 100 milligrams of THC before they even begin to feel relief from their pain.

Tolerance is generally dependent upon your biology and body size.

After a few months of taking 5 to 10 milligrams of THC every morning, you might discover that the same dose doesn't give you the same effects that it used to. Your body has adjusted to the dose, and you may need to increase it to get the same high that you used to get.

I love coffee. I love the taste, and I love how it makes me feel. Awake, alert, focused. My moderate daily coffee intake is two double espressos, and I know that's a lot, but some days I drink four double espressos to power through long workdays and stressful deadlines. Eventually, I overdo it too many days in a row, and then I don't feel the lovely effects of coffee anymore; I've ruined my tolerance. I don't feel good after two double espressos; I don't feel awake, alert, or focused. To reset my body and get back to feeling good with a normal serving of caffeine, I buckle down and skip coffee for a week. I suffer through the withdrawal headache and nap a lot. Then, one glorious morning, I sip a single espresso and feel amazing.

We have the same control over our cannabis tolerance. Cut back on edibles, smoking, and vaping for a few days as much as you can, then go back to your starting dose. You may feel some irritability for a day or two, and your pain might flare up, but it does not take long to reset your cannabis tolerance to a lower dose.

To make sure my tolerance doesn't get out of control, I make sure to use moderation every day. Vaping concentrates make my tolerance go up, so I vape concentrates only when my sciatic nerve pain is at least a five on the pain scale. If I wake up feeling good, I'll skip my morning dose of cannabis oil, just to keep my tolerance in check.

HOW DOES IT FEEL TO GET HIGH?

My mother came to visit me at work in the dispensary. She looked at plants, smelled jars of marijuana, and met patients who came in to buy medicine.

"Want to try a gummy? Five milligrams will feel good, and you won't get high," I said.

"Oh, no." She didn't consider it for a second.

"Fine," I said. "Mexican for dinner? Margaritas?"

"Yes," she said, just as quickly. "I could use a margarita."

My mother has never tried cannabis. But she knows from experience exactly how a margarita will affect her. Even though one drink will make her loopier than 5 milligrams, she sticks with the poison she knows.

Many people have never tried marijuana, and they are nervous about the first time. What does it feel like? Will I hallucinate? Will I lose control? Will I embarrass myself? It might be a little scary to try getting high, but the most important thing to remember is that getting high is fun. It feels good. And a marijuana high can be milder than some highs we know from the hospital, the dentist, or the pharmacy.

"It felt like I inhaled a yoga class." A patient was talking about her experience with a particular strain, but it's the perfect description of the euphoria of a marijuana high. You know you're high when you feel like you just sat up from the most restorative, euphoric yoga class you've ever had.

Cannabis is psychoactive but not psychedelic. When high, you still feel like yourself, just a more relaxed and happier version of yourself. Being high is mind altering, but not in an extreme way. Marijuana doesn't cause a loss of balance, control, or inhibitions like a pitcher of margaritas can inspire. There are no blackouts or hangovers. Hallucinations are possible, but only if you really overdo it.

There are so many strains and so many different kinds of cannabis products, it's no surprise that there are so many different kinds of highs. Indica and sativa are just the beginning.

Different Kinds of High

JUST A LITTLE HIGH: Sometimes, a mild high is just what the doctor ordered. Social events, yoga class, and even a trip to Target are more fun with a little bit of a buzz. If you can do it after two glasses of wine, you can do it with a mild high. One-to-one (or 1:1) strains, with equal and balanced amounts of THC and CBD, are ideal for a mild high. Stick with strains under 10 percent THC and edibles with 10 milligrams of THC.

I DON'T FEEL HIGH, BUT I DO FEEL GOOD: CBD doesn't make us high, but it does make us feel better, and for some people, feeling better—less pain, anxiety, depression, and stress—feels like getting high because it feels so good. Choosing a low-THC, high-CBD strain relieves pain and improves mood without a euphoric high. Strains with less than 5 percent THC or edibles with less than 5 milligrams of THC are all appropriate cannabis medicine for times when we don't want to get too high, but we do want to feel better.

HAPPY AND GIGGLY HIGH: We often describe the psychoactive effect of marijuana as a mood enhancer, but another way to say it is that getting high is a pleasure enhancer. Food tastes better, music sounds better, funny things are funnier, sex feels better. Yoga is better and meditation is easier. For a social, fun high we don't want to get too high, so stick to strains around 10 to 20 percent THC for smoking and vaping and 20 milligrams of THC for edibles. Check out hybrid strains so you get the best of both worlds—a cerebral, fun high with a bit of a body high to relax.

WRITE A POEM HIGH: Artists have been getting high to produce beautiful music, art, and books since the dawn of time. Cannabis is a creativity boost and increases focus while it reduces depression and anxiety—the perfect cocktail for productive, creative work. The cerebral high of a sativa strain is why these strains are so popular at the dispensary. But the thing is, too much of a sativa can increase anxiety, which kills creativity. For most people, the ideal artistic edible dose is 10 to 20 milligrams of THC for the high, with 5 to 10 milligrams of CBD to moderate anxiety. For smoking or vaping, look for strains and concentrates with lots of citrusy and sweet-smelling terpenes like limonene and pinene.

SO RELAXED I CAN'T GET OFF THE COUCH HIGH: The harder our brains and bodies work, the more they need rest. Adrenaline and stress hormones power us through stress-filled days, weeks, and months, but eventually our bodies need to unplug, turn off, rest. When I feel like this, I take a hot bath, rub cannabis-infused cream into my feet and legs and neck and shoulders, then cue up the Netflix, light scented candles, and curl up with a cashmere blanket and a high-THC indica strain that smells like earth, hops, and cloves. (Granddaddy Purps is my favorite indica strain to relax with.) The high is not in my head like it is with a creative sativa. The high is in my body as the muscles relax and stress dissolves away. Getting to the fridge feels like a monumental task, but I always get there. I go to bed early, sleep eight or nine hours, and wake up feeling like I took a vacation.

The First-High Checklist

1. **DECIDE WHO YOU WANT TO GET HIGH WITH.** If you feel nervous about your first high, make sure to do it with people you feel comfortable with and who make you laugh. Ideally, it would be someone who has gotten high before, but two first-timers can also handle it. It's also fine to do it alone, because you are going to start with a low dosage and go slowly and responsibly.

2. **DECIDE WHAT METHOD.** Smoke, vape, or eat. If you eat, eat 10 milligrams of THC—and no more!—and keep in mind that it takes up to ninety minutes to kick in. Choose an edible with both THC and CBD for the most medicinal high. If you vape for your first high, get a prefilled cartridge and battery. The budtender will show you how to put it together. Take it one inhalation at a time, just like smoking, but wait at least thirty minutes between each inhalation. Cartridges come in many different THC:CBD ratios. The budtender can advise you, or you can simply ask for what you want.

3. **PLAN YOUR SNACKS.** Before you get high, get yourself a glass of water and make sure you have great things to nibble on. Don't think about gluten or calories or carbs. This is the moment for good chocolate and your favorite treats. Think about taste and flavor, because once you get high, that's all you're going to care about.

4. **GET COMFORTABLE.** Yoga pants, pajama pants, or no pants at all. Turn on your favorite music and turn down the lights. You should be finished with the day's responsibilities and ready to relax in bed.

5. **CONSIDER YOUR ACTIVITIES.** Try creative, artistic pursuits like coloring books, knitting, sewing, and painting. Or binge-watch episodes of your favorite show. One that makes you laugh is a good choice. One caveat: Getting high slows down our short-term memory, so reading while high is generally no fun.

6. **RELAX AND ENJOY YOUR HIGH.** Notice your body relaxing and unwinding. Enjoy the mood boost and let yourself have a good time.

Recommended Marijuana for Different Styles of Yoga

Yoga reduces stress, increases relaxation, and makes us feel and look great. So does marijuana. And getting high before a yoga class exponentially boosts the benefits of both. But we have to match the right kind of marijuana to the right kind of yoga. A stimulating sativa doesn't help us sink into a deep yin practice, and a strong indica might lay us out flat on our mats in an Ashtanga class.

To time your high to your yoga, eat the edible an hour before the class begins, or take a tincture a half hour before class, or inhale a few minutes before. Choose a 1:1 THC/CBD strain or edible/tincture for a mild high and maximum stress reduction.

As a special treat to release tension, I sometimes rub a cannabis-infused cream into my neck and shoulders before class.

ASHTANGA/VINYASA/HOT/POWER/ANUSARA—A sweaty flow class with lots of movement is best suited to energetic sativa-dominant strains. Take a small dose to stay mindful of your movements and breathing. Try Ghost Train Haze or Island Sweet Skunk.

HATHA—This classic yoga style is a little bit vigorous and a little bit relaxing, just like a good hybrid, such as Blue Dream or Pineapple Express.

IYENGAR—With an intense focus on alignment and props, Iyengar yoga is not for the stoned. Choose CBD-rich marijuana to lift your mood and reduce pain, while keeping you clearheaded to focus on your alignment. Look for Harlequin, Cannatonic, and other CBD-rich strains.

KUNDALINI—Once, a friend and I smoked a joint before a Kundalini class. When the chanting and breathing exercises started, we got the giggles so badly we had to leave the room. Wear white, be prepared to flow a little, and don't get too high. Stick with a 1:1 THC/CBD.

YIN/RESTORATIVE—When you spend an hour lying on the floor, wrapped in blankets, and not moving, a strong indica is the best choice. Restorative yoga classes are meant to reduce stress and increase relaxation, just like a good indica.

THINGS TO REMEMBER

- THC gets us high and also makes us feel better. CBD makes us feel better without getting us high.

- A balanced amount of THC and CBD helps reduce pain and treat more conditions than THC alone.

- Dispensaries display marijuana by strain name and indica or sativa, but what we really want to see are the potency lab testing results for cannabinoids and terpenes.

- Terpenes determine if marijuana is indica or sativa. Edibles have very few terpenes, so edibles are not indica or sativa, just THC and CBD.

- To choose the correct strain, decide if you want THC, CBD, or equal amounts of both. Then choose indica or sativa.

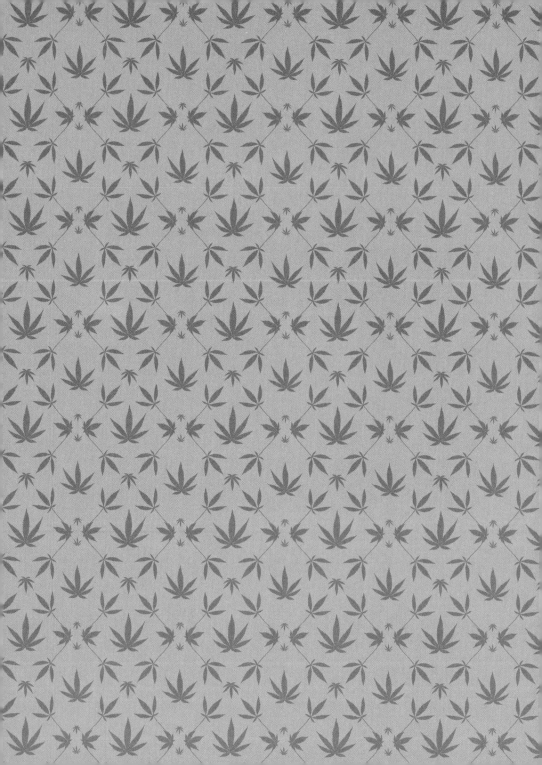

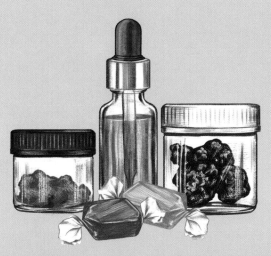

Part Three

BUYING CANNABIS—
WHAT TO ASK FOR,
WHAT TO LOOK FOR

When experienced marijuana users walk into a dispensary for the first time, they all usually say the same thing: "I feel like a kid in a candy store." But for someone who has never tried it before, shopping for marijuana can be overwhelming. This section of the book provides all you need to know to shop intelligently for cannabis and to leave with what you want.

WAYS TO TAKE CANNABIS MEDICINE

Just a few short years ago, dispensaries offered marijuana flower and poorly made marijuana-infused candy. That was pretty much it. But now, we can buy transdermal patches, mouth sprays, and suppositories in dispensaries. Cannabis medicine makers are constantly developing new products, and they're focused on making medicine that not only gets us high, but also makes us feel better.

Remember that a psychoactive high depends on the amount of THC in a single dose, but the high also depends on how we consume that THC. We can eat, smoke, vape, or rub into our skin 10 milligrams of THC, but the effects and the highs will be different for each. Smoking 10 milligrams of THC gets us really high. Eating 10 milligrams is a mild high, and 10 milligrams of hand cream won't get us high at all.

Mode of administration is the unsexy term for how medicine enters the body. Inhaling marijuana is one mode of administration. Eating it is another. But we can also consume marijuana with a sublingual, rectal, transdermal, or topical application. Each one has its own benefits, onset, and duration of effect. Some are more effective than others, and some are more fun. But it's important to know them so you know which mode of administration is best for you. A cannabis-infused cream isn't going to touch anxiety, and a 50-milligram suppository is too much THC and will increase anxiety.

INHALING is the most well-known way to consume cannabis, and one of the most popular. Smoking or vaping marijuana has the fastest onset of effects, which means we get high quickly—usually within about fifteen minutes—and it can last from two to four hours. It also means we can easily control how high we get.

When marijuana is inhaled, about 10 to 15 percent of the THC, CBD, and other medicinal compounds are absorbed and used by the body. Because inhalation avoids the digestive system, it is especially effective for anyone dealing with nausea or digestion issues. We inhale by either smoking or vaping, and we can smoke or vape cannabis flowers as well as cannabis concentrates.

Recommended for anyone who wants to feel the effects quickly and control the intensity of the high.

EDIBLES are a popular method of consuming cannabis, because while not everyone likes to smoke, just about everyone likes to eat. When cannabinoids pass through the digestive system, they are released into the bloodstream and lock into receptors in the

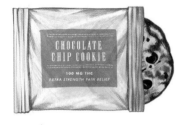

endocannabinoid system; we feel high, but not right away. It can take an hour or two for the THC in a brownie to produce a euphoric effect, but that effect will last much longer than the effects of inhaling. On average, an edible dose lasts twice as long as an inhaled dose, so the high can last from four to eight hours. It's not easy to adjust the dose of an edible because it takes so long for them to begin working, so it's important to remember to start low and take it slow. If you have never tried a marijuana edible before, start with 5 to 10 milligrams of THC. Don't take more until you know how 5 to 10 milligrams affects you.

Eating an edible has a bit more bioavailability than inhalation; around 20 percent of the medicine will be absorbed and used by the body. There is no difference between 10 milligrams of THC in a cookie and 10 milligrams of THC in a gummy. Eat the one that tastes good to you.

Recommended for anyone looking for a longer effect and who can wait an hour or two before effects are felt. Edibles include capsules, food, and drinks.

SUBLINGUALS are marijuana in liquid form that are absorbed by placing a few drops under the tongue. When cannabis is absorbed in the mouth rather than swallowed, the body absorbs more of the milligrams because the digestive system doesn't get involved. Cannabinoids that are absorbed in the mouth don't pass through the liver as edibles do. The liver reduces the number of milligrams that get into the bloodstream and get us high. Almost 50 percent of the cannabinoids in a sublingual are absorbed by the body. A sublingual application will take ten to twenty minutes for effects to be felt, and effects continue to rise for about four hours until a peak is reached, which means pain relief lasts for hours. It's also a great mode of administration for anyone who has trouble swallowing. When my brother is in the middle of a seizure, it's a sublingual application that I reach for, either a tincture or a spray.

Recommended for nonsmokers, anyone with digestive issues, or anyone who can't wait for an edible to work. Sublingual products are oils, tinctures, hard candy, mints, lozenges, and breath sprays. Anything that goes in the mouth but isn't swallowed.

RECTAL APPLICATIONS are cannabis-infused suppositories. They are the most efficient way to consume marijuana. As the suppository melts—it is most often made of cocoa butter—the cannabinoids are absorbed by veins in the rectum and quickly enter the bloodstream, which means the effects are felt much faster than with an edible. And because the marijuana doesn't pass through the stomach and liver, cannabinoids are not wasted on the first-pass digestion, which means more marijuana is available for the body.

Fifty to seventy percent of the cannabinoids in a suppository are absorbed and used by the body, and the effects of a marijuana suppository are felt for four to eight hours. The best thing about a marijuana-infused suppository is that the high is much milder than with any other method of consuming marijuana. Eating 50 milligrams of THC might send you into a 12-hour power nap, but a 50-milligram suppository is simply relaxing.

Recommended for anyone with digestive issues or a lot of pain. For now, suppositories are only available in a few states. But you can easily make them yourself, in whatever dose you prefer (see page 190 for the recipe).

TRANSDERMAL APPLICATION means that cannabis enters the bloodstream through the skin. Transdermal patches, similar to nicotine or opioid patches, allow cannabinoids to sink through the skin and into the bloodstream and we get high. Very high, as I discovered when I applied my first patch to my arm. It sent me on a dog walk that lasted for hours because I couldn't find my way home. After that, I began recommending for patients to cut the patches in half. The next time I tried a patch, I had a throbbing broken toe, and it almost immediately eliminated the pain and kept it at bay all day. Transdermal patches are calorie-free, the effects kick in quickly—faster than with edibles but not as fast as with smoking/vaping—and last for six to eight hours.

Recommended for anyone who needs a strong dose that lasts a long time. We can't make transdermal patches at home; we have to buy them in a medical or recreational dispensary. They are available in THC, CBD, THC/CBD, and other options, so you can find the cannabinoids that work for you.

TOPICALS are applied to the skin but do not enter the bloodstream, so we don't get high. Instead, cannabinoids and terpenes lock into the endocannabinoid system receptors that are located in the skin. Considering how effective cannabis is at healing the rest of our bodies, we shouldn't be surprised at the miraculous things it does for our complexion. Creams, lotions, and oils infused with cannabis relieve pain and inflammation without a psychoactive high. Pain relief can be felt within an hour of applying a topical and can last for several hours. Arthritis responds wonderfully to marijuana topicals, since the cannabinoids and terpenes reduce both inflammation and pain. Sore muscles and nerve pain are also reduced with cannabis creams. Topicals work for more than just acne, psoriasis, dermatitis, and eczema. Rubbing marijuana oil on your temples can help relieve a headache. We aren't as concerned about the number of milligrams per dose in topicals, because there is no high.

Recommended for localized muscle pain, arthritis, and other inflammation issues. Topical products include skin creams, lotions, salves, and balms. Topicals usually either improve the condition of the skin itself or relieve pain. THCA and CBDA are just as effective, if not more so, at reducing inflammation and relieving pain, so look for topicals that contain a whole range of cannabinoids, not just THC. Patients report anywhere from one to four hours of pain relief from topical applications.

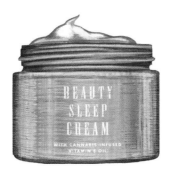

THE LEGAL RULES
OF CANNABIS

My mom's friend Nancy had lung cancer. She spent hours on the internet researching marijuana treatments. She was packing her bags for California when she checked in with me. She knew she needed marijuana oil, and she knew it would be expensive. She asked if I had any other tips for her trip.

"Don't buy anything that hasn't been lab tested," I said. "Make sure it's pesticide-free. And look for oil that says *whole plant* or *flower run*. Those are more potent."

"Flower run," Nancy repeated, scribbling notes. "Now, do I want THC or CBD?"

"Both. Get grams of each or buy oil that has both."

This went on for another twenty minutes, and she sounded determined when she hung up. A week later my mom called. "Well, it didn't go like she thought it would."

"What happened?" I asked.

"She drove halfway across the country and ended up buying oil from a man in a parking lot," my mom said. "But she said it looks like pictures she's seen online."

It's very easy to get a medical marijuana card in California, if you are a California resident. But a Missouri resident will walk out of a California doctor's office disappointed and empty handed. In the parking lot of the doctor's office, a seventy-year-old woman with terminal cancer who just lost her last hope is an easy mark. A polite young man convinced her that she didn't need the dispensary, state regulations, or lab testing. His marijuana oil was just as good, and lucky for her, he just so happened to have the 60 grams she was looking for—right there in the trunk of his car. She never asked why he didn't have anything better to do at eleven a.m. on a weekday. She didn't ask why his oil wasn't sold in a dispensary. She was desperate and dying and had cash in her hand, so she bought her miracle cure and went home, breaking federal laws every time she and her husband crossed a state line. Nancy's illegal, untested cannabis oil did not reduce her pain. Many terminal cancer patients successfully use cannabis oil to help them sleep and eat during their final days, but it's cruel to make it so difficult and risky to obtain.

A well-regulated legal market protects medical marijuana patients and forces legal marijuana producers to make safe, high-quality medicine. The black market makes no such promises. Heavy doses of harmful pesticides, mold, fungus, and dangerous solvents can turn lifesaving medicine into life-threatening poison. It is vitally important for every marijuana user to understand how effective and safe marijuana medicine is made, so they can protect themselves from unscrupulous salespeople and recognize the difference between low- and high-quality medicine in the dispensary.

Even though medical marijuana is legal in most states, it is still illegal at the federal level. In a state with legal medical marijuana laws, the police and prosecutors will not arrest or charge anyone who follows the laws of that state, but the DEA (Drug Enforcement Administration) makes no such promises. In recent years, the federal government and states with legal medical marijuana programs have reached an uneasy truce. As long as cannabis cultivators, producers, and retailers follow state law and act as responsible businesses, the DEA will leave them alone. Responsible cannabis companies promise to stay off federal and public property, not cross state lines, not sell product to minors, not launder money, not commit other crimes, and not sell their product on the black market.

Thankfully, state laws are changing quickly, even if the federal government is slow to act. And as new medical marijuana programs develop, state by state, lawmakers and cannabis companies learn from past mistakes and get better at what they do. Older, more mature cannabis markets refine and adapt old rules and adopt new rules all the time. After several harvests tested positive for dangerous pesticides, many states adopted laws that prevented cultivators from using those pesticides on cannabis plants. After Maureen Dowd, a widely read *New York Times* columnist, got too high on a chocolate bar and wrote a chilling description of the experience, labeling and potency rules changed. Colorado was the great recreational experiment when it became the first state to allow any adult to buy cannabis, for any reason, and now that more states are becoming recreational/adult-use states, the new rules reflect the lessons that were learned in the mountains.

Here's the thing, though. Cannabis production and sales are not allowed by the federal government, so the cannabis industry is not regulated by the federal government. There are no FDA requirements or standards to follow, no food safety standards, and no federal inspectors. The coffee you drank at breakfast and the burger you ate for lunch were more regulated and checked for safety than the cookie you got at the dispensary. Just a few generations ago, you couldn't trust the food at the grocery store to not make you sick or kill you, so federal agencies were created to make sure the food supply and medications are disease-free, but the cannabis industry is basically winging it.

The good news is that sometimes capitalism does exactly what it's supposed to do. The legal cannabis industry is growing faster than any other industry, ever. The dot-com boom was a soft rainfall compared to the hurricane of money to be made in cannabis, and as each year passes, cannabis companies are developing their own standards and best practices to create the most effective and innovative products. The products and strains on the shelves today are so much better than they were five years ago, and that process and growth is not going to stop anytime soon.

With so little regulation and so much money to be made, the best and the brightest are now jumping into cannabis, and they have big pocketbooks. Titans of industry are throwing millions of dollars into cannabis research because they see the billions to be made. So, even without federal safety regulation or supervision, the market is driving itself to create, improve, and perfect cannabis medicine.

In some states it is legal to grow your own cannabis plants at home. In others, it is not. To make sure you follow the rules of your state, look up the regulations online. There is a government website that explains the rules and regulations of cannabis in your state, and a quick Google search should bring you right to it. There are some basic rules that apply to everyone, no matter where you live, and they apply to both medical and recreational users.

IT IS ILLEGAL TO:

- Cross state lines with cannabis, no matter how you cross (walking or by bike, car, plane, etc.)

- Fly or drive from one recreational/adult-use state to another with cannabis

- Send cannabis through the mail

- Resell cannabis purchased in a dispensary

- Give cannabis to minors

- Use cannabis in public

- Use cannabis while driving (In most states—even where it is legal—you can get a ticket for having cannabis within reach of the driver's seat in the car. On the drive home, store your purchases in the trunk or the back seat of the car.)

To stay on the right side of the law, buy medical marijuana in a dispensary, put it in your trunk, take it straight home, and don't share it, especially with children. Treat your marijuana like your prescriptions, alcohol, and bleach. Keep it secure, up and away from curious little hands, like you do with the medicine cabinet, liquor cabinet, and cleaning cabinet.

When traveling, you are allowed to purchase cannabis in any recreational/adult-use state. For a patient with a medical card, a few states do offer reciprocity—they accept medical marijuana cards from other states. Nevada allows this. If you go to Vegas with your medical marijuana card from Massachusetts or Minnesota, you can shop at medical dispensaries in Vegas.

If you are traveling to a state that does not have medical reciprocity with your home state or is not a recreational/adult-use state, you should not bring your cannabis medicine with you.

Every state requires that all cannabis be sold from dispensaries. Dispensaries are a strange hybrid of pharmacy and candy store, and like pharmacies, they have lots of security cameras and a computer system that tracks every single gram of medicine, just like the pharmacy tracks every pill. But the pharmacy doesn't have BOGO half-off sales of their medications, or "spend $100 and get a free pre-roll" sale, and many dispensaries do. Dispensaries are retail stores and everyone can buy whatever they want, so producers make products and packaging look as appealing as possible.

There are cannabis pills available at dispensaries, but in a weird quirk, capsules are the least popular products at the dispensary. My take on the reason for this is that by the time patients seeking medical marijuana have come to a dispensary, they've taken hundreds of pills that just made them feel sicker and didn't relieve their pain. The last thing they want to get at a dispensary are pills, because pills have done nothing but fail them. Chocolate bars, on the other hand, have never disappointed anyone.

SHOPPING FOR MARIJUANA IN THE TWENTY-FIRST CENTURY

Years ago, when I lived in New York, a neighbor gave me a pager number. Whenever I called it, Junior would appear. Junior was a happy, smiling Jamaican man who spent all day driving around the city, delivering marijuana. I would hop into his 2002 gold Taurus and ride around the block while we talked about the weather and traffic and he told me funny stories about his kids. I would tuck a hundred dollars into his glove compartment, and he would slip a couple of small zipper storage bags, stuffed with marijuana flower, into my hand. He was the best marijuana dealer I've ever met. Dependable, polite, and he delivered to Brooklyn on Sundays.

I still miss delivery, but Junior only had one strain. He didn't know if it was an indica or a sativa. He didn't have potency testing, and no one checked the flowers for mold. He didn't have lotions or gummies or transdermal patches. There's another marijuana delivery service in New York, and only famous people are given the number. They have cannabis-infused lip balm and edibles, but they don't have lab testing.

Retail is the best part of legal marijuana. Stores, with regular business hours and pretty displays of flowers, concentrates, edibles, sublinguals, and topicals.

The main difference between a medical and a recreational dispensary is that a medical dispensary requires a buyer to be a registered medical marijuana patient in the state, with a state-issued patient ID. A recreational dispensary only requires that you be over the age of twenty-one, with ID to prove it. Both have a full selection of cannabis products, but the medical-only stores tend to stock more medicinally beneficial products like capsules and topicals, while recreational stores focus on getting high with lots of options. In most states, prices and taxes are lower for medical patients, so to keep costs down, a medical card is a good idea. Most dispensaries only accept cash. Health insurance does not yet cover medical marijuana, but I have faith that it will one day.

If a dispensary has neon signs and Bob Marley posters in the window, they are looking for a younger, recreational crowd, which means they stock their store with a lot of products made specifically for getting high and may not have the more medicinal products that focus on pain relief.

Dispensaries that cater to a medical crowd take themselves more seriously. The receptionist might be wearing a lab coat. They do not have a pot leaf on the door. These stores are stocked with lots of products that are created for medical patients, and the staff is well educated and more able to help beginner patients. Be aware of the image a dispensary is trying to project, and go to the one that speaks to you.

When you get to the dispensary for the first time, don't pass judgment on its location. Dispensaries require extra security cameras, vaults, and more-secure deliveries than other stores, so it's difficult to open a dispensary in some retail locations. They are doing the best they can with the laws they have to abide by, like not being located a certain distance from a school or church, and some regulations require them to be in an industrial part of town. Don't go anywhere that makes you feel unsafe, but don't needlessly worry either. My favorite dispensary in Denver has handsome security guards who escort you to your car, even though it's located in a Target parking lot in a safe neighborhood. At the dispensary, you are as safe as you are at the bank or the pharmacy.

Good dispensaries are clean, well-lit places, staffed by budtenders with expertise in cannabis and a well-developed sense of compassion. They get to know you and learn your tastes and preferences. Because they understand cannabis medicine so well, they are able to stock their shelves with the best, most effective products, and they don't stock anything they don't believe in.

Dispensaries that cater to a medical crowd take themselves more seriously.

Average dispensaries focus on sales and trinkets. The staff isn't as passionate, knowledgeable, or well paid. No one has curated the selections—the customer can't tell which products are great and which are not. Average dispensaries are fine if you know exactly what you're looking for, but beginner patients are going to feel lost and overwhelmed.

Bad dispensaries are cheap. That's it. That's all they offer. The staff can't help you, and they don't have lab testing results. If you know exactly what you want and they have it on sale, go for it, but know that it probably hasn't been tested for mold or pesticides. Bad dispensaries focus solely on THC and don't have CBD-rich flowers and edibles.

TIPS FOR CHOOSING A DISPENSARY

- Dispensaries are reviewed online by customers, just like any other business. Review websites like Google and Yelp can also tell you everything you need to know. Apps and websites like Weedmaps and Leafly focus on marijuana dispensaries and can tell you which take credit cards, which have lab testing, and which strains are available that day.

- Look for dispensaries with lots of CBD strains and products, not just THC. Good dispensaries have marijuana with full cannabinoid profiles. If the dispensary only stocks high-THC strains, they're only interested in selling recreational marijuana. There is no difference between medical and recreational strains of cannabis; Granddaddy Purps can be used just for fun, or it can be used to relieve pain. But good dispensaries stock plenty of CBD-rich strains so patients have options.

- Good dispensaries display the potency testing for each strain of flower. They don't sell anything that tested positive for mold or pesticides, and they display the test results where you can see them easily as you shop. If they don't test their medicine at all, it means they don't care about their medicine and you shouldn't either.

- Good dispensaries do not dispense medical advice. They don't tell you to stop taking your prescription medication without telling your doctor. If you find that with cannabis you don't need your prescription anymore, talk to your doctor about reducing your dosage.

- Some dispensaries are pricier than others, but don't let price be your deciding factor. The less expensive cannabis is generally less effective, so saving money will, to some extent, lessen the effectiveness of the medicine.

Walking into the Dispensary

From the moment you get out of your car in the parking lot at the dispensary, you are on camera. This is for your own safety and the safety of the dispensary. As soon as you step inside a medical-only dispensary, someone will ask for your ID and medical card. At a recreational dispensary, they will only require your ID. Neither type of dispensary will let you stay without identification, so make sure you have it before you leave the house.

When you arrive, tell them this is your first time. Some budtenders are better with new patients than others, and telling them right away that you're new to this gives them a chance to get the staff person best suited for new patients. Plus, many dispensaries give a discount or special treat to first-time patients. After they check your ID, they will either lead you into the store to meet with a budtender or they will park you in the waiting room to wait your turn. If you wait, use this time to look over the menu.

Dispensary menus list the products they have available for sale that day. Like the farmers' market, not every strain is available in every dispensary, simply because there are hundreds of strains to choose from, and dispensaries can't carry every single one of them. And depending on the garden and the dispensary, they may not have all their usual options available at all times. Remember, cannabis is a plant, and buying cannabis medicine is like buying produce. The season and growing cycle dictate what is available and what they're out of, so check the menu every time you shop at the dispensary.

A budtender will come get you from the waiting room and

lead you to the counter to choose your medicine. Most dispensaries are set up like jewelry stores, with a glass case of products on display. Tell the budtender what condition, disease, or pain you want to treat and whether you want to smoke, vape, or eat your medicine, or apply it to your skin. All day long, that budtender talks to patients just like you, so they know which creams are working well for arthritis and which creams don't seem to get the job done. Ask for their opinion, just like asking the waiter about the special of the day. Dispensary staff have tasted the edibles and smoked the flowers, so they know what tastes good and what doesn't.

The budtender is your key factor for a successful shopping experience.

Dispensaries train their budtenders to instill as much knowledge about the medicine as possible. Like everything else in the marijuana industry, there is no standard or regulation for training or education for dispensary staff, so good dispensaries train their staff on their own.

Even at a great dispensary, there are not-so-great budtenders, and the person helping you is the most important factor for a successful marijuana shopping experience. Keep an open mind. I've met tattooed youngsters behind the counter who were more helpful than pharmacists, so don't judge them on looks alone. Good budtenders aren't stoned. Okay, this may not be true. I've met several kids behind the counter, giggly and red-eyed, but they knew what they were talking about, and they listened well and took care of patients with professionalism and kindness.

There are a few tricks to knowing whether you have a good budtender. Good budtenders don't touch the medicine with their bare hands. They don't push the special of the day or whatever their manager told them to sell today. They answer your questions without making you feel silly for asking them. Good budtenders build a relationship with you, to the point where you wonder if you should buy them a Christmas gift.

Find a budtender who cares about you.

Bad budtenders don't remember you, even though they've waited on you four times. Bad budtenders don't know the difference between a cannabinoid and a terpene, and they don't want to take the time to answer your questions, because they don't know the answer. Or, they think they're an expert, but they simply can't be bothered to explain the basics. A bad budtender pushes you to buy medicine that you don't want or need, and they rush you out the door before you have a chance to ask about test results and potency. They will tell you that "everything we have is good," but they can't tell you the difference among them.

A good budtender might be covered in piercings and neon hair dye, and a bad budtender might be wearing a lab coat and sensible shoes. Give everyone a chance, but keep looking until you find a budtender who understands you.

Buy Flower

If you decide to smoke or vape marijuana flower, choose the strain you want, then decide how much you want to buy. Flower is sold by the gram and the ounce.

Some dispensaries also sell *trim* or *shake*. Trim is the trimmings from the cannabis plant—leaves and flowers. Trim is for cooking, not inhaling. Shake is pure cannabis flower; it's just been broken down or ground up from its flower bud shape. Trim and shake are much less expensive than cannabis flower and are a good option for making your own edibles at home.

When sampling a new strain, buy a gram of cannabis flower—that's about one joint's worth of flower. That way, if you don't like it, you didn't waste money on it. If you know you like a strain, buy more at a time to save a few dollars. When I go to the dispensary to stock up, I buy a quarter ounce of a sativa, a quarter of an indica, and a quarter of a 1:1. These quarters usually last me a month of light smoking on a daily basis.

⅛ ounce = 3.5 grams = "eighth"   ½ ounce = 14 grams = half ounce

¼ ounce = 7 grams = "quarter"   1 ounce = 28 grams = ounce

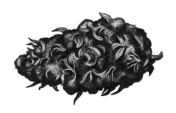

Buy Concentrates

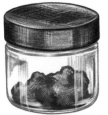

Vaping, which we'll get into soon, involves buying a cannabis concentrate or buying a vape cartridge. Concentrates are prepackaged, sold by the gram, and go by names that describe their textures—wax, shatter, or live resin.

Vape pen cartridges are prefilled with concentrate oil, measured by milligrams, and more powerful than flower. Most cartridges have 250, 500, or 1,000 milligrams of oil. Cartridges with more oil are more expensive, but they last a lot longer.

Buy Edibles

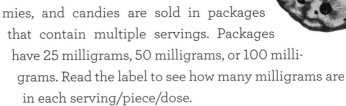

Edibles are sold by the package and measured by milligrams of cannabis they contain. Some candy bars are wrapped individually, but mints, gummies, and candies are sold in packages that contain multiple servings. Packages have 25 milligrams, 50 milligrams, or 100 milligrams. Read the label to see how many milligrams are in each serving/piece/dose.

SAMPLE DISPENSARY MENU

Flower

All flower available in pre-rolls ($12), ⅛ ounce ($50), or ¼ ounce ($95)

Sativa

Durban Poison (19% THC)
Island Sweet Skunk (17% THC, 0.5% CBD)
Sour Diesel (24% THC, 0.3% CBD)
Lemon Haze (21% THC)

Indica

Granddaddy Purps (21% THC, 0.2% CBD)
Kosher Kush (27% THC)
LA Confidential (17% THC)
Grape Ape (16% THC)

Hybrid

Blue Dream (16% THC)
White Widow (17% THC)
Girl Scout Cookies (15% THC)
Cinderella 99 (23% THC)

THC/CBD Strains

Cannatonic (8% THC, 6% CBD) (hybrid)
Pennywise (11% THC, 10% CBD) (indica)
Harlequin (10% THC, 12% CBD) (sativa)

Shake

Tangerine Haze (sativa, 20% THC)— ½ ounce—$100
Cherry Pie (hybrid, 18% THC)— ½ ounce—$100

Edibles

Betty's Bombdiggity Brownies— 100 mg THC/100 mg CBD total (10 servings per package)—$50
Tincture (cherry or lemon flavor)— 30 mg THC/300 mg CBD total (30 servings per bottle)—$70
CannaMints—100 mg THC total (10 servings per package)—$25

Topicals

Mary's Medicinals Transdermal Patch—15 mg THC/CBD— $15 (3 for $35)
Cannacream Pain Rub—100 mg THC total—$30

Concentrate

Disposable vape pen (500 mg)—$30
Vape Pen Cartridges
THC (1,000 mg)—$60
CBD (1,000 mg)—$60
1:1 THC/CBD (1,000 mg)—$60
Shatter
Strawberry Cough (hybrid)—$50
OG Kush (indica)—$50
Live Resin
Green Crack (sativa)—$60
Granddaddy Purps (indica)—$60

Dispensary Pricing

When a state creates a new medical marijuana program and brand-new dispensaries open their doors to first-time patients, prices for cannabis medicine are sky-high. As the program matures and the number of patients increases, prices come down, but it can still cost a significant amount of money to medicate with cannabis on a regular basis. Health insurance doesn't cover the cost, and it would cost thousands of dollars to try out every product on the shelves, so how do we know which products are worth buying and which are not?

I am not a bargain hunter, but I do shop wisely. When I buy clothes, I think about how often I'm going to wear a particular item of clothing, and I divide that number by the price. A $500 evening gown? My cost per wear is going to be huge because I will rarely wear it. A $200 cashmere sweater that I'll wear three times a week, six months of the year, for five years? Worth it. I'd rather buy a $200 sweater that lasts five years than buy a $30 sweater that falls apart in a single season.

When I buy infused cannabis products, I look at the cost per milligram to find the best deal. If a package of marijuana gummies costs twenty dollars and has 100 milligrams, it means I'm paying twenty cents per milligram. So if there is a package of gummies with 100 milligrams for twenty dollars and a package of hard candies with 50 milligrams for fifteen dollars, the gummies are the better choice because they cost twenty cents per milligram, while the candy costs 30 cents a milligram.

Make sure to compare apples to apples and oranges to oranges. All food is absorbed by the body in the same way. The

TIPS TO SAVE MONEY AT THE DISPENSARY

- **Buy in bulk.** The price per milligram comes down when you buy more, so if you know something works for you, stock up and save a few dollars. You can store your cannabis flower for months in an airtight glass jar, and it will continue to cure and improve its flavor.

- **Check the cost per milligram.** Just divide the price by the number of milligrams ($20/100 milligrams = 20 cents).

- **To save money on cannabis flower, ask the budtender if they have any shake.** Shake is cannabis flower that has fallen off the stem and now looks ground up, rather than remaining a whole bud. Shake should have almost the same potency as regular flower; it's just not as pretty so it doesn't fetch top dollar.

- **Make your own edibles and topicals at home, with concentrates.** Concentrated cannabis, such as CO_2 oil, is a lot more potent than cannabis flower, and every single milligram of THC and CBD is infused into the edible, unlike flower, which loses almost half of its potency when extracted into butter, oil, or alcohol. If I buy 3.5 grams of flower to make a jar of pain cream, it will cost around $50, and I'll get around 350 milligrams in my cream when I'm finished. If I buy 1 gram of CO_2 oil, it will also cost around $50, but my cream will have more than 700 milligrams, so I can make twice as much cream for the same amount of money.

high is the same and the effects last the same amount of time, so it doesn't matter which cookie we eat—we only care about how much cannabis is in the cookie. Tincture, on the other hand, is absorbed in the mouth and is more bioavailable, which means we need to consume fewer milligrams for the same effects. Comparing 100 milligrams of tincture to 100 milligrams of an edible isn't fair, because you'll get more bang for your buck with the tincture.

Topical creams, lotions, salves, and oils may have expensive ingredients that drive up the cost. Fancy marketing and packaging can all make cannabis medicine cost more, too. Many dispensaries offer discounts for veterans, and also check for a senior discount.

BUDTENDER FAQS

Every good budtender I know loves his or her job. They like to answer questions and be creative. They like to learn from their customers and to listen as much as advise. Here are some of our most frequently asked questions. I'm answering them in the first person, because while the questions are common, the answers are going to vary in real life based on the person asking and the person answering.

Q: How do I find my ideal dosage?
A: Studies have shown that inhaling a cannabis blend of 10 milligrams of THC and 10 milligrams of CBD is the most medicinally beneficial daily dose of cannabis we can take,

so if you're not sure where to start, start there. I consider an "ideal dosage" to be a regular dosage of cannabis—perhaps daily—that allows you to live your life with little to no pain and stress. Ten milligrams of THC is a mild high, especially when combined with 10 milligrams of CBD. This small, daily dose relieves pain, prevents dementia, boosts mood, and relieves anxiety and depression. If 10 milligrams of THC feels too high for you, try 5 milligrams of THC in the morning and 5 milligrams of THC at night. And, of course, there are different ways to take that dosage. I take my ideal dose by rubbing a single drop of cannabis oil on my gums. It has no calories, no smoke, and works as a sublingual, so the cannabis is absorbed into my body without passing through the digestive system, which means it works faster than an edible. It lasts several hours, and it's just right for me. To do this, I buy CO_2 oil, packaged in an oral syringe, allowing me to squeeze out just a drop at a time. If you're interested in this intake method, ask your budtender for CO_2-extracted cannabis oil. If they don't have it, ask for suggestions for the next best thing. Fair warning: Cannabis oil does not taste good. If it gets on your tongue, a swallow of juice or a bite of something flavorful should wash the taste away.

Q: How can I relieve my fibromyalgia/chronic pain/nerve pain?

A: When your pain level creeps up the chart and becomes debilitating, you may need more THC and CBD than your regular daily dose. Moderate to strong pain may need 20 milligrams for beginners, and some patients need even more than that. Nerve pain is fierce and difficult to treat without very high doses of THC. I've met people with cerebral palsy who have seen amazing benefits with cannabis, but they didn't find relief until they started taking 100 milligrams or more a day of THC. I would recommend 20-plus milligrams of THC and 20-plus milligrams of CBD, taken by inhalation, edibles, sublingual, or topical, depending on location of pain and severity.

Q: I'd like to sleep better, solidly, and wake up refreshed.
A: For most people, a couple of inhalations of a heavy indica strain is enough to get to sleep. CBN is a minor cannabinoid that acts as a strong sedative, and sometimes I find CBN-specific products, like transdermal patches, at the dispensary. Ask your budtender if they have any CBN-rich products. For me, edibles get me to sleep—always. But everyone is different.

I recommend a strain with 20 milligrams of THC, low-to-no CBD. Look for indica strains and products with CBN and myrcene. Take it in any form, but remember how long it takes for each to become effective. Edibles can take forty-five minutes to an hour, so account for that time before you crawl into bed. And remember that generally speaking, a high-THC blend is not that conducive to reading, if that's what you're used to doing before falling asleep.

Q: I'd like to improve my appetite after dealing with illness, and my partner wants to resist food cravings that are not on his food plan. Is there something for each of us?
A: People living with HIV, AIDS, and cancer struggle to eat enough to maintain a healthy weight. Wasting syndrome and anorexia are qualifying conditions in many states, and for

anyone who needs to boost their appetite, THC is the solution. One of my favorite cancer patients used to tell me that one inhalation was enough to get rid of his nausea, and a second inhalation was enough to make him hungry enough to eat. And then some of us struggle to stay at a healthy weight because our appetite is stronger than our body needs, and we want to reduce our hunger. For us, CBD is our hero. Most days, 10 milligrams of CBD is enough to keep me on my food plan, but some days I need an extra dose for the willpower to resist pizza.

I recommend 10 milligrams of THC to increase appetite or 10 milligrams of CBD to reduce appetite, taken by inhalation or as a sublingual; avoid edibles.

Q: I'd like to help my partner with her digestion issues due to Crohn's disease.

A: Inhaling marijuana can be a lifesaver for people with Crohn's disease because it provides immediate relief of nausea. When a new patient comes to the dispensary with digestive troubles, I like to start them off with a THC vape pen or sublingual tinctures to avoid the digestive system. Then, I steer them toward the indica strains. I recommend starting with 10 milligrams of THC and 10 milligrams of CBD taken by inhalation. Edibles are to be avoided due to the nausea associated with food.

Q: What can I take for menstruation/menopause symptoms?

A: Medicating with marijuana when Aunt Flo comes to town can relieve bad moods and abdominal pain before they start. I have severe cramps, so one day a month, I eat a high-THC edible and take a long nap, and then I smoke a CBD-rich strain throughout the day for a few days to manage my abdominal pain. You might need more or less. Consider layering your cannabis medicine—inhale for immediate relief while eating an edible for slower-acting, longer-lasting relief. I recommend a 20-milligram-THC/20-milligram-CBD blend. For severe cramps, a 1:1 THC/CBD suppository is very effective, and a THC tincture or edibles at night increase relaxation, relieve stress, and promote good sleep.

Your own ideal dose should address most menopause symptoms. Keep a vape pen handy for quick inhalations to relieve acute symptoms like night sweats and mood swings. THC lowers body temperature and will keep you from sweating through the sheets.

Q: I work at a creative job and would like to use cannabis to enhance my performance.

A: Sometimes taking the edge off at work will not only allow you to make it through the day, but it just may give you new ideas and a fresh perspective. Obviously, you should not smoke in the office—don't overdo it, smell like weed, or be careless. Bring a vape pen to discreetly medicate during the day. Sativa is the route to go at work, as it keeps you sharp. Choose a 1:1 THC/CBD strain to reduce stress and boost creativity, or choose a CBD-only strain to stay clear-headed and focused. If your job is chronically stressful and anxiety-inducing, consider keeping a package of low-dose cannabis-infused edibles—such as 5-milligram mints—in your desk.

Q: I would like to consider other ways than psychopharmacology to address my anxiety and depression.

A: If you are taking any kind of prescription medication, you must, I repeat MUST, discuss your desire or intention to change medication with your doctor. That said, I have many customers who have found relief from their depression and anxiety symptoms with cannabis. For many people, the commonly prescribed ideal dose of 10 milligrams of THC and 10 milligrams of CBD is also the right dose for mood management. Too much THC often increases anxiety, so keep that THC dose low. CBD is a powerful antidepressant, so look for CBD strains and edibles to increase your happy without getting high.

Q: Is there a role cannabis can play in my regular exercise workout and recovery?

A: I quit roller derby after two practices because I hurt myself the first time I fell down. The women that stick with roller derby amaze me with their athleticism and their bruises. When women push their bodies that hard, they need a recovery plan, and cannabis can help. Out-of-shape exercisers are athletes, too. Walking a mile can be a great achievement, but it can also make you sore as hell if you're starting out with a new exercise routine. If you are working hard, treat yourself like an athlete, no matter how fast or far you go. Rub a cannabis-infused pain cream into sore feet, ankles, knees, hips, backs, shoulders, and neck. I recommend a low THC/high CBD strain before and during workouts, and the ideal dose (10 THC/10 CBD) for recovery. Take it by inhalation or sublingual tincture to avoid extra calories in edibles, plus a topical pain cream to rub into sore muscles.

Q: I've heard cannabis can be a sexual aid, too. Is that true?

A: Cannabis is thought to be an aphrodisiac, and we can use it in a few different ways to live our best sex life. Use a vape pen for an inhalation or two of an indica, body-high blend of 10-milligram-THC/10-milligram-CBD strain for relaxation and a good mood, or plan ahead and share an edible for dessert, so the effects are felt by the time you get to the bedroom. When you get there, use some cannabis-infused massage oil and lubricant for extra tingle.

Q: I don't want to get high around my kids, but I wish I could manage the feelings of overwhelming frustration I sometimes have around them.

A: You're right. You do not want to be high around your kids, and you want to be ready to handle any emergency that might come up. But a high-CBD blend of sativa allows you to care for yourself and your kids and still keep everyone safe. I wish I could have given this advice to the mom I saw outside of the coffee shop one day, who, after loading her temper-tantrum-throwing children into their car seats, shut the last car door, slid down the back of the car, lit a cigarette, and cried. Parenting has gotten more stressful, more time-consuming, and more labor intensive. Mommies are often on edge and need the relaxation of cannabis more than anyone. CBD-rich vape pens and edibles keep Mommy calm and happy and *not high*, so she can handle any emergency that comes her way. I recommend 5-milligram-THC/10-plus-milligram CBD taken by vape pen or edibles.

Q: What can I use to help with dementia, tremors, and seizures?

A: THC is wonderful for dementia, tremors, and Parkinson's symptoms in adult patients, but dosing is critical. The problem is that older patients are more sensitive to the negative effects of THC (anxiety and short-term memory loss), but serious tremors or pain may require a higher dose of THC, or more frequent doses throughout the day. I know one woman with Parkinson's who couldn't calm her tremors until she started eating a 5-milligram-THC/5-milligram-CBD candy every two hours throughout the day. A 20-milligram candy increased her anxiety, but when she split the dose in half, she was able to find the sweet spot that relieved her tremors without increasing her anxiety.

Most of the seizure patients whom I've met, including the children, need a dose of THC with their CBD to keep seizures at bay. Scientists are still studying the effects of cannabis on the brain, but they have found that both THC and CBD are important for brain health.

Many medical marijuana patients, particularly the oldest and the youngest, don't inhale their medicine; they eat edibles or take sublingual oils. But the ideal dose doesn't apply to children because their bodies and endocannabinoid systems are immature. With kids and elders subject to seizures, we dose by weight. To figure out a daily dose, start with 0.5 milligram of cannabis per pound of body weight (for example, a 40-pound child would take 20 milligrams). Divide that daily amount into three to four doses taken four to six hours apart. Some do fine with this, and some need 1 to 2 milligrams per pound of body weight before their overactive brains are calm. Some children do well with very low-THC, high-CBD cannabis, while others need more THC and use a 1:1 THC/CBD cannabis medicine.

GROW YOUR OWN PLANTS

Not everyone is allowed to grow their own cannabis plants, but many people are legally allowed to grow their own medicine at home. Cannabis is called weed for a reason, because cannabis plants grow like weeds. A little light, soil, water, and plant food are all it takes to grow your own plants and save money at the dispensary.

If you live in a state that allows you to grow cannabis plants, the dispensaries in your town will sell baby plants, called clones, that you can take home and grow yourself. Dispensaries also have seeds, if you want to start from scratch. Seeds and clones are available in different strains, so you can grow your favorite indica, sativa, or hybrid strains.

If you know how to grow a tomato plant, you know how to grow a cannabis plant. You can even use the same plant food. If you buy a clone in the spring and plant it outside in your backyard, by fall you could have more than a pound of marijuana. Just make sure the plant is somewhere where children (or deer, or adults) can't get to it. If you build an indoor garden with a tent and lights, you can be Mother Nature and you can harvest your plants year-round.

If you have never tried to keep a plant alive, pick up a book by Jorge Cervantes to learn everything you need to know about cultivating cannabis plants at home.

Start very low, go very slow, and keep experimenting until you find what works. Do this in consultation with a doctor and do not change prescribed medication in any way without your doctor's assistance and knowledge.

TIPS FOR THROWING A CANNABIS PARTY

Marijuana parties are so much more fun than alcohol parties. When we trade in our wine bottles for marijuana, we still get to relax, have fun, and enjoy ourselves. And the next day, we're not hungover. We're well rested and hydrated.

When I host a marijuana party, I take a few steps to make sure everyone feels comfortable and has a good time. I make sure I have good weed, great snacks, and fun things to do.

- Invite fun, laid-back people, and warn guests ahead of time that you'll be getting high, not tipsy. If you or your guests are cannabis newbies, keep the group intimate and familiar.

- Have options. Plan for both edibles and inhalation. Not everyone can eat edibles, and not everyone enjoys inhaling.

- Serve 5 to 10 milligrams of edibles as soon as guests arrive, so they feel the effects when the party gets going, not when they're going home. Keep the doses small so guests can choose a dose that fits their tolerance. Some people prefer

5 milligrams of THC while others prefer 20 milligrams of THC. Just like with alcohol, guests should be prepared to call a car service to get home if they've had too much.

- Choose hybrid strains for smoking and vaping. Avoid a full indica strain, or at least one person will fall asleep on the couch. If you serve a full sativa, someone else is going to feel anxious and uncomfortable. I speak from experience.

- Have something for everyone. Serve CBD-only edible options for anyone who doesn't want to get high, and have a 1:1 THC/CBD strain on hand for anyone who likes to inhale a mild high.

- Set up a water station. Dry mouth is a side effect of using marijuana, so fill a pitcher with ice water and muddled fruit, and keep it filled. Juice, soda, and iced tea are also good choices.

- The open-kitchen floor plan was designed for the munchies. Your happy guests will be looking for flavor, so serve something delicious, and bring your guests into the kitchen to cook with you. Get your Julia on and get fancy, or keep it simple with fresh-from-the-oven cookies and a pitcher of ice-cold milk. And, of course, make sure the edibles are clearly marked and kept separate from the munchies.

- If serving edibles, do not serve virgin forms of the edibles, or people will get confused. If the edible is a truffle, keep the munchies non-truffle and do not serve anything that can be confused with a truffle.

- Plan a creative activity. Set up easels for a painting party or make crafts. Nothing too complicated, but use lots of color. I know one particular group of suburban mommies who get together every fall to smoke joints and make elaborate Halloween costumes for their children. The cannabis-inspired outfits are a big hit at the Trunk-or-Treat gatherings, and one of them always wins best costume.

THINGS TO REMEMBER

- How we consume marijuana is just as important as which kind of marijuana we use. Choose the best mode of administration for you—inhaling, eating, sublingual, rectal, transdermal, or topical.

- Stay legal. Yes, there are ways to obtain cannabis illegally, but you won't know what you're getting and how good it is. And then there's the law. Best to follow it.

- If you don't see what you're looking for, ask your budtender. Many dispensaries keep their products behind the counter and under glass, so we can't always read packaging labels ourselves like we can at the grocery store.

- A good budtender is as valuable as a good hairstylist. When you find one, hang on to them.

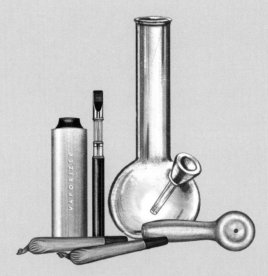

Part Four

INHALING CANNABIS—FAST AND EFFICIENT

The next big question about cannabis: Do I want to smoke it? Even if you know in your bones you don't want to smoke, don't skip this section. A lot of patients come to the dispensary convinced they don't want to inhale. So they try edibles, creams, and tinctures and they find some relief from their symptoms and pain, but eventually, they all reconsider and start asking about smoking and vaping. In this chapter, you'll find out why.

SMOKING CANNABIS IS HEALTHIER THAN EATING A CHEESEBURGER

The idea of inhaling medicinal smoke may sound strange, but it can be a really pleasant experience if you want it to be. Cultures and civilizations have created entire ceremonies to celebrate the smoking of medicinal herbs.

Cigarette smoke and cannabis smoke contain many of the same dangerous and carcinogenic compounds, yet studies have shown that chronic marijuana smoking (a joint a day for over twenty years) does not cause lung damage or impart a higher risk of cancer.* A pack of cigarettes a day can kill us; we all know that. But a joint a day can actually improve lung tissue

---

*Mark J. Pletcher, Eric Vittinghoff, Ravi Kalhan, Joshua T. Richman, Monika Safford, Stephen Sidney, Feng Ying Lin, Stefan G. Kertesz, "Association Between Marijuana Exposure and Pulmonary Function Over 20 Years," *JAMA Internal Medicine* 307, no. 2 (January 2012): 173–181.

and make us healthier. The theory is that the medicinal cannabinoids and terpenes that are inhaled in the cannabis smoke are so powerfully anti-inflammatory, they counteract the mild inflammatory damage of smoke and tar.

Smoking cannabis is not totally harmless, however. Be aware that smoking does increase the risk of bronchitis and increases the amount of mucus in the throat, which can cause a wet smoker's cough, which is not chronic—it ceases when smoking ceases. Smoke is an irritant, which is why our bodies make mucus. Cannabis smoke is considered a mild irritant.

The best reason to smoke cannabis is that the effects are felt immediately.

In dispensaries, 40 to 60 percent of all sales are for raw cannabis flower. Some patients use the flower to make edibles, but most are smoking it. Smoking is the least-expensive way to use cannabis on a regular basis, which makes it a popular option because cannabis medicine is not inexpensive.

But the best reason to smoke cannabis is that the effects of smoking are felt immediately, and one or two inhalations are enough to feel happy and relaxed within seconds. If you eat cannabis in a brownie, it can take up to an hour before pain relief comes, but inhaling cannabis provides immediate pain relief. When smoking cannabis, the high lasts for an hour or two, and we can control exactly how high we get, inhalation by inhalation.

The Quality of Cannabis Flower

At the upscale florist in the nice neighborhood, I spend $100 for a dozen roses. At the gas station down the street, a dozen roses is available for $19.99. When I place the bouquets side by side, the reason for spending extra money becomes clear. The expensive roses are much more beautiful and last a lot longer than the gas station roses.

The same is true of cannabis flowers. High-quality cannabis looks, smells, and smokes much better than low-quality flower. High-quality cannabis is more potent, so the medicine is more effective and worth the extra cost. The best cannabis flower is organic and free of pesticides and mold, with the lab results to prove it. It's easy to see the difference while shopping in the dispensary, if you know what to look for.

High-quality flowers smell good, and the odor is strong because the flower is coated with trichomes. This coating appears like a sparkly layer on the flower, and it holds terpenes—the medicinal compounds that give cannabis its smell. Citrus, sweet, hops, skunk—whatever the dominant odor of that particular strain, it should smell strongly of it. Poorly dried and cured cannabis flower smells like hay or grass. Curing is when the smell really comes together, so if that step of the process is skipped, the cannabis won't smell good.

The best flowers are hand trimmed, not machine trimmed. When cannabis plants are harvested, the flower needs to be trimmed. The flower buds have small sugar leaves that need to be removed before we consume them. Growers can either hire human beings to trim the plants, or they can get a machine to do the work. Of course people cost more, but the final result is much, much better. Trim machines chop up flowers and remove the coating of trichomes. Sometimes, the biggest difference between high-quality flower and bad flower is the trim job.

Evidence of the quality of cannabis flower can also be seen in the ash. After you smoke it, it burns down and turns to ash. If the ash is bright white, it means the cannabis plant was properly "flushed" and the flower does not contain any pesticides, fertilizers, or plant foods. "Flushing" occurs during the last two weeks of growth, when the plant is watered with plain water and no plant food, fertilizers, or pesticides are used. This washes away the salts and additives that build up in the soil and roots of the plant. If the ash of a joint or pipe is gray, the plant was flushed a little bit, and if the ash is dark and black, the cannabis was not flushed at all. This won't cause you any immediate harm, but it would be wise not to buy from that supplier again.

After the cannabis flowers are cut from the plants, dried, and trimmed, they need to spend some quality time in an airtight glass jar to cure. Curing is the process of slowly removing the last of the moisture from the flower. Tobacco is cured for maximum flavor, too.

The best flowers are bright and colorful, with hints of pink, purple, blue, and orange hairs tucked among the bright green flower buds. Bad flower is a dull greenish brown, with no colorful hairs.

Properly dried and cured marijuana flowers are big and dense and sticky, without being too wet or too dry. Low-quality buds are not dense and are either too wet to smoke or so dry they crumble into dust. If you want to see what prizeworthy flowers look like, Instagram has lots of photos of beautiful artis-anal, organic cannabis flowers. Mid-quality flowers are not bad medicine; they just aren't Instagram worthy.

Any variety of cannabis can be well cultivated, well har-vested, and pesticide-free. Blue Dream can be the best flower in the dispensary or it can be the worst, depending on how well that particular plant was grown. The budtender knows which strains look great and which don't, so ask them for their opinion. Smell the jars or examine the flowers through the packaging if you can.

The amount of THC and CBD in the cannabis does affect how the flower looks. THC makes plants and flowers look prettier—more color, more sparkle. CBD makes cannabis flower look a little more rustic than the blue-ribbon perfection of THC plants and flowers. CBD-rich strains smell as lovely as THC-rich strains, and the same steps are required to create high-quality flower—flushed, dried, trimmed, and cured properly—but CBD strains will always struggle to win any beauty contest.

Most dispensaries price flower according to quality, with the worst being deeply discounted and the best priced as high as the market will bear.

I cannot tell the difference between boxed wine and a $200 bottle. To me, all beer tastes the same. But I would walk across fire to get my hands on Kona coffee beans. I can tell the dif-ference between true Jamaican Blue Mountain coffee and the knock-off blends. I am as discerning about marijuana as I am about coffee; I am as sensitive to the differences in marijuana strains as I am to the difference between light roast and dark roast. For me, paying a few dollars more for the best flower in the dispensary is worth it.

But if every cannabis strain tastes the same and you can't tell which strain is the boxed wine and which is the $200 bottle, don't think of yourself as a failed weed snob. Think of yourself as an economical cannabis user, because you can buy the medium-priced marijuana and get the same effects. As long as you shop at a dispensary with a very good reputation for quality goods, you can buy the less expensive stuff. Just don't go to a low-quality dispensary and buy the cheapest stuff.

HOW TO JUDGE A CANNABIS FLOWER			
	HIGH QUALITY	MID QUALITY	LOW/DISCOUNT QUALITY
SMELL	Strong and good	Weak	Grass/hay/ chemical
TRICHOMES	Disco-ball sparkle	Glitter sparkle	No sparkle at all
TRIM	Hand trimmed	Machine trimmed	Machine trimmed
FLUSH	White ash	Light-gray ash	Dark/black ash
CURE	More than 30 days	Less than 30 days	None
MOISTURE	Balanced and sticky	Too wet or too dry	Too wet or too dry
COLOR	Bright green	Dull green	Brown
INSTAGRAM	Worthy	Maybe Facebook	Hide from social media
PRICE	Saks	Anthropologie	Target

Smoking Tools

Dispensaries stock all the marijuana supplies you could ever need, including vaporizers, rolling papers, cleaning solutions, storage containers, and glass pipes in a variety of sizes, shapes, and colors. We can also order smoking and vaping tools online, because it is legal to ship them across state lines. There are dozens and dozens of options, each with its own style, so it's easy to find one that fits your look and lifestyle.

- **LIGHTER.** Get a disposable full-sized lighter. Don't use a reusable lighter—it will affect the taste negatively. Matches are fine, but may affect flavor.

- **GRINDER.** Get a small manual coffee grinder–type device that breaks up marijuana buds into a coarsely ground shake that is rolled into papers for joints or packed into bowls to smoke. You can break up buds with your fingers, but they will leave a sticky residue on your hands that is difficult to wash off.

- **AIRTIGHT GLASS JAR.** Your marijuana flower is best stored in an airtight glass jar. The jar will continue curing the flowers for several months until you are ready to smoke them, which results in a better smoke and flavor. The buds will dry out if you leave them in the plastic packaging or in a container that is not airtight. Keep each strain in its own jar. Do not smoke seeds, stems, or leaves. Properly stored, flowers will continue to cure and stay fresh for months, or even years.

- **PIPE.** The most popular way to smoke marijuana is with a pipe, and glass is the best pipe material. The more expensive glass pieces are handblown by local artists, and the less expensive pieces are imported from Chinese factories. 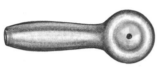 Save your pennies and buy handblown glass. It will last much longer and look more beautiful than the imported glass. Each pipe has a different-sized bowl, where we lightly pack the coarsely ground flower. Choose a larger bowl for sharing with friends, and a smaller bowl like a chillum or one-hitter for medicating by yourself. Be sure to choose a pipe that has at least 6 inches between your face and the bowl. Once, I bought the cutest little glass pipe shaped like an elephant. The bowl was on the elephant's back and you inhaled from the trunk, but the pipe was so tiny that every time I touched a flame to the bowl I practically set my eyebrows on fire.

- **ROLLING PAPERS.** You can buy pre-rolled joints at the dispensary, or you can roll your own. "Empty cones" are rolling papers already rolled around a paper filter. Simply stuff the cone with shake and smoke. All rolling papers are basically the same, so choose the size you prefer. 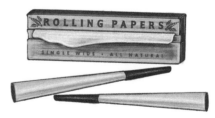 Flavored papers are also an option. They are akin to flavored coffee.

- **BONG.** Bongs are simply water pipes, and they come in a variety of sizes. Save the larger ones for social gatherings and get a small one for personal use. Water pipes tend to offer smoother, bigger inhalations than regular pipes.

- **ASHTRAY.** Smoking creates ash, and you need a place to put it. Obviously, anything can work for this, from a pretty seashell (properly dried!) to an old plate.

- **FRESHENING-UP KIT.** Smoking smells; there's no way around it. If you medicate by smoking flower, you need a freshening-up kit to stay clean and smell-free. Eye drops for red eyes, hand wipes to clean the smell from your fingers, gum or mints to freshen your breath, lip balm, and a touch of perfume will keep you from smelling like a hippie. Stash a bottle of water in your go-bag, too. Dry mouth is a prevalent side effect of smoking cannabis.

- **AIRFLOW.** If you smoke marijuana in your home, the smell will linger, but not like cigarette smoke. Marijuana smoke will fill the room with its distinctive smell, but an open window and a fan clears up the problem in no time. Prop the fan in the window outward, so the fan sucks the smoke from the room.

How to Smoke a Joint

If you choose to smoke a joint for your first high, a pre-rolled joint is a good option. Dispensaries sell pre-rolls that are made of a filter and very thin paper, and contain up to a gram of marijuana. The filter tip works just like a cigarette.

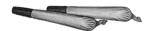

1. With a lighter, apply the flame to the twisted end (not the filter) and gently inhale. Don't hold the flame to the paper for too long; just touch the flame to the paper and let your inhale pull the flame into the flower.

2. Once you inhale a lungful of smoke, release it immediately. The cannabinoids and terpenes have already entered your body through the lung tissue, and holding in the smoke for longer won't get you any higher. After one or two inhalations, gently stub out the burning end of the joint in an ashtray and save it for later. You can relight the joint over and over again until it's gone. You do not need to, nor should you, smoke the whole thing at once.

3. Notice how you feel. Take a deep breath, relax your shoulders, and focus on your body. One of the best reasons to smoke cannabis is fast-acting pain relief, so become aware of your pain levels and how they change in the next few minutes. If you chose a sativa, you might perk up a bit, like when your morning coffee kicks in. If you chose an indica, you may feel like lying down is the best idea you've ever had. If you chose a high-CBD strain, your pain should decrease quickly.

4. If you feel good, and about twenty minutes have passed, and you want to try another inhalation, go for it. For some symptoms and conditions, one or two inhalations is enough medicine. Others need a lot more before the relief comes. If you need more, smoke more. You'll figure out how much to smoke and how often, but right now we're just getting familiar with the process of medicating. Wait ten minutes between inhalations to avoid getting too high.

You might not feel anything, and that's okay. Not everybody gets high the first time, and nobody knows exactly why. Our bodies produce cannabinoids, and some people may naturally have higher or lower levels of natural cannabinoids and receptors that affect the body's ability to absorb cannabinoids from the plant. Some people try marijuana and they feel high and love it immediately, and other people try marijuana and either nothing happens or they don't enjoy it at all. Don't give up if the first time doesn't go well. Try again with a smaller dose.

VAPING FOR DISCRETION

The worst thing about smoking marijuana is the smoke. It smells—and most people recognize the smell, which can make smokers self-conscious. When you smoke, you also create ash, which can be messy. Vaporizers, on the other hand, are clean, discreet, and elegant. Vaping gives us all the benefits of smoking, with none of the smoke. Vaping is the same process as smoking—inhaling cannabinoids and terpenes into the lungs—but without the combustion of fire. Vaporizers and vape pens are discreet and can be used indoors. They look like they produce smoke, but that cloud is just vapor, and it does not smell like marijuana.

Dispensaries sell vaporizers. They are available at every price point, and for the most part, you get what you pay for. Some vaporizers have extremely sophisticated and practical designs, and some are cheaply made and will break after a few uses. Some are better for larger doses, while some are better for on the go. I'll go into detail on the varieties, but there are two main types.

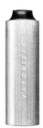

PORTABLE OR HANDHELD VAPORIZERS are easy to carry in a purse or bag. They run on batteries and need to be charged like a cell phone. Like a glass pipe, they have a small bowl for flower, which heats up at the touch of a button. The heated bowl releases cannabinoids and terpenes into a vapor that is inhaled like smoke, but doesn't smell like smoke.

TABLETOP VAPORIZERS are large instruments that are meant to be used at home. With some machines, vapor fills a bag of air that is inhaled. Other machines release vapor when the user inhales from a plastic tube. These are great machines for sharing with friends.

What to Vape: Cannabis Concentrates

There are two different forms of cannabis to choose from to put in your vape: flower or concentrates. Cannabis flower can be smoked or vaped as is, but concentrates—a fairly new evolution of cannabis—are specifically designed to be vaporized.

Concentrates are made by separating the medicinal compounds of marijuana from the plant matter. When marijuana flowers are turned into concentrates, several grams of cannabis flower are converted into 1 gram of cannabis concentrate, creating a powerful medical substance that takes the form of a sticky goo called *wax*, a fragile solid called *shatter*, or oil.

Five years ago, when I was forty, my age was the great divide between consumers of flower or concentrates. Younger-than-forty patients vaped concentrates, while anyone older than forty smoked flower. At the time, vape pens hadn't taken off in popularity yet, so the tiny jars of goo—and the blow torches required to heat them—didn't appeal to older and more sophisticated crowds. Now, with more advanced and reliable vaporizers that make it easy to use concentrates, they're appealing to every age of consumer.

The last few years have seen handheld vaporizers and disposable vape pens explode in popularity as an easy, elegant way to vape. The simplest vape pens are nothing more than a battery and cartridge. You screw the cartridge on to the battery and inhale gently on the mouthpiece. When the cartridge is empty, it is thrown away and a new one is screwed on. Dispensaries are stocked with cartridges in different strains and flavors. I use vape pens in the car with my mother when she's driving and she never knows. Vape pens are ideal for people who need to medicate discreetly.

Cannabis flower is 20 percent medicinal compounds like cannabinoids and terpenes, and 80 percent plant matter that is not medicine. When we smoke marijuana, we inhale the plant matter, which doesn't help us, but it doesn't harm, either. Concentrates, on the other hand, are anywhere from 50 to 90 percent medicinal compounds. A tiny dose, a literal dab of goo, contains enough medicine to relieve pain for hours. Vaping concentrates have the same effect as smoking or vaping flower: We feel high almost immediately, and it lasts for an hour or two.

Concentrates require trial and error. Marijuana flower smokers have learned the hard way that concentrates are much stronger than anything they have tried before. If you decide to try a concentrate, take one inhalation. Just one. Wait a full hour before taking another. Notice how you feel and how it affects you. If you ignore my advice and decide to take two hits, find a glass of water and a place to lie down.

BHO (BUTANE HASH OIL)—Cannabis producers use butane (the same fluid that's in a lighter) to extract the medicinal compounds from the plant matter, then they remove the butane from the oil. Most of the products in dispensaries are made with butane hash oil. The texture of a butane concentrate determines its name. Wax, shatter, crumble—all defined on page 126.

CO_2 OIL—CO_2 oil is magic. It has all the medicinal compounds of cannabis with none of the plant matter. The oil is packaged in an oral syringe, so to use it we simply squeeze out a drop or two at a time. We have to be careful with this oil, because we can easily get too high with just an extra drop. CO_2 oil can be vaped or eaten.

VAPE PEN CARTRIDGES—Cartridges are pre-filled with potent marijuana oil—CO_2 oil. Dispensaries stock cartridges in a variety of potencies and strains, and they are simply screwed on to a small, rechargeable battery. Take an inhalation anytime you need a shot of pain relief. Vape pens hold hundreds of inhalations, can last for weeks, and are easy to carry around in a bag.

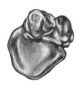

WAX—Wax is a soft, solid chunk of concentrate, similar to hash. A dab tool or skewer can be used to pull off a small dab of wax that is then loaded into a vaporizer.

SHATTER—The only difference between wax and shatter is texture. Shatter is more solid and will break into pieces.

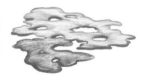

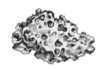

CRUMBLE—Simply a drier version of wax. Crumble can be picked up with your fingers without sticking to your skin. Sugar, sap, budder, and honeycomb are other names of concentrates that are defined by their texture.

LIVE RESIN—Most concentrates are made with dry flowers, but live resin is made with frozen flowers, which saves more of the terpenes and gives live resin a better flavor and smell than other concentrates.

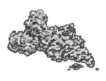

PAINT THINNER/RSO—RSO stands for Rick Simpson oil. The internet is full of recipes for making marijuana oil at home using paint thinner as a solvent. Paint thinner is not safe for consumption, and this oil should not be eaten, vaped, or smoked.

KIEF/DRY SIFT—The oldest method for concentrating marijuana is to gently rub marijuana flowers over screens to separate the trichomes from the rest of the plant matter. Trichomes, the sparkly stuff that covers the flowers, contain most of the cannabinoids and terpenes in the marijuana plant. When we use a grinder to break up marijuana flower, kief collects in the bottom of the grinder.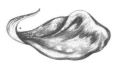

ROSIN—Rosin is the newest way to extract without a solvent and is the easiest concentrate to make at home. Marijuana flower is simply pressed with heat, which releases medicated oil. A hair straightener and parchment paper are the only tools needed to literally press oil out of the flower. The oil is scraped off the paper and vaped in a vaporizer.

BUBBLE HASH—Also known as water hash, ice hash, or solventless hash. Water is used to separate the medicinal compounds from the plant matter by agitating marijuana in ice water. Bubble hash can be smoked, vaped, or cooked into edibles.

Different Types of Vaporizers and How to Use Them

There are dozens of vaporizers in different styles and sizes. Some can be used to vape flower, some are used for concentrates, and some can be used for both. You don't ever need a lighter or an ashtray, and there is no smell when you vape.

VAPE PENS—Disposable vape pen cartridges are easy to use, don't smell, and require zero cleanup. Pens made up of a battery 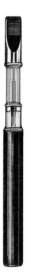 and a cartridge require charging via a basic USB charger. Then you simply put the mouthpiece in your mouth and inhale. Some pens need to be turned on before inhaling by pressing a button a few times. When the cartridge runs out of oil, simply unscrew it, dispose of it, and buy a new cartridge. Cartridges are available in THC, CBD, 1:1, indica, sativa, and hybrid.

If you inhale on your pen and it doesn't work, it may be clogged. Blast the cartridge with some hot air from a hair dryer. The oil might just be too cold and solid, and a little heat warms it up and gets it moving again. Pens can leak, too, so keep yours in a container when you carry it around.

HANDHELD VAPORIZERS—If vape pens are beginner vapes, then handheld/portable vaporizers are intermediate-level vaporizers. They can be used with flower or concentrate, and while they're bigger than a pen, they still fit in a clutch, so you can take your vaporizer anywhere you go. Vapor does not smell like smoke does, so they are perfect for discretion. Handheld vaporizers are bigger and more powerful, with stronger batteries, so they can go longer without being charged, reloaded, or cleaned.

I love my Firefly vaporizer. It feels solid and expensive and obsessively designed. Like any portable vaporizer, there is a small bowl to hold the concentrate or flower and heat it until it vaporizes. I use a dab tool, similar to the tool manicurists use on my cuticles, to scoop a tiny amount—a dab—of concentrate, and I smear it into the bowl of the vaporizer. I snap on the lid, hit the button, watch the coils heat up, and inhale the vapor. I release the button, exhale, and I'm finished. When I vape concentrated marijuana, one inhalation is more than enough for me to feel high and relaxed. But the vaporizer also vapes cannabis flower, so I can buy anything at the dispensary and vape it in my Firefly. Because concentrates are more concentrated, vaping flower isn't as potent as vaping shatter or wax, so I take two or three inhalations of vaped flower.

The Firefly is one of the most expensive vaporizers, at $300 or more—I saved my pennies for months to buy it—but it certainly isn't the only portable vaporizer on the market. The Pax vaporizer is another high-end, well-designed device, and other portable vaporizers are available at different price points. Dispensaries sell vaporizers, so ask your budtender to help you pick out the right one for you. They are also available online, of course.

TABLETOP VAPORIZERS—These are advanced-level vaporizers and are best suited for groups of people or anyone who needs high doses for significant pain. There are two versions. One is hookah-style, where vapor is inhaled through a tube. The other version fills a clear plastic bag with vapor, like a balloon. Tabletop vaporizers can be used with cannabis flower or concentrate, but they aren't portable and are for home use primarily.

MARIJUANA IS A LOT STRONGER THAN IT WAS BEFORE

Every time I'm with a middle-aged friend trying marijuana again after years of responsible child-rearing, they get way too high. Every time. I warn them, I try to stop them, and they do it anyway. When friends came to visit me in the mountains, they toured the dispensary and garden, marveled at marijuana-infused tea bags and lemon bars, and immediately took too much.

"Slow down, it's a lot stronger than it was in the nineties. And you're forty now."

"Oh, I'll be fine." They take three inhalations in a row, without waiting to see how one or two will affect them. And suddenly they're way too stoned.

I can tell when they've had too much because they stop talking. They no longer make eye contact or seem to acknowledge that anyone is there at all—but their own hands have become so fascinating they can't stop staring at them. When this happens, I know I've got about an hour before they come around and can have a normal conversation again, so I take away the marijuana, get them a big bottle of water, and look for the best tacos or doughnuts (usually both) I can find.

Slow down. It's a lot stronger than it was in the nineties—or any year before that.

The cannabis flower in legal dispensaries is more potent than the marijuana we smoked in college, no matter how old we are. (It's also a lot more expensive.) There is a lot more THC in a single joint now, so to get comfortably high, we need to smoke a lot less of it than we used to.

In the sixties and seventies, baby boomers smoked marijuana that grew wild, outdoors, without genetic manipulation. THC was around 5 to 10 percent, much lower than the 20 to 30 percent potency we see in the dispensary today.

In the eighties and nineties, when illegal marijuana cultivation moved indoors to avoid detection, growers were able to exert more control over the growing process. Better lighting, nutrients, and growing conditions boost the potency of the flowers on the plant. A healthy, well-grown plant produces much more marijuana, of a much higher quality, than a poorly grown plant. Potency increased from 5 to 10 percent THC to 10 to 20 percent THC during the end of the twentieth century because of indoor cultivation and better plant genetics, but it was the legal marijuana market of the twenty-first century that really boosted THC potency levels to new heights.

The legal market is competitive, and cannabis cultivators are constantly striving to increase the THC potency of their plants, because that's what the market demands. A lot of patients think that buying higher-potency THC is a bargain, so they look for the highest THC potency they can find. Now we all know, because we've been reading this book, that the amount of THC in a cannabis flower isn't nearly as important as the balance of all the cannabinoids and terpenes in cannabis, but most other users don't know this yet. To meet that demand for higher THC, careful breeding and lab testing by cultivators, now legal, has boosted THC potency levels up to 30 percent in a few select strains. This isn't a bad thing; it just means we need to consume less flower when we get high. Ten percent THC means I need two or three inhalations to feel high. Thirty percent THC means I just need one inhalation to get high. Don't be afraid of high potency; just make sure to consume less to avoid anxiety.

THINGS TO REMEMBER

- Don't buy marijuana based on just THC. A 15 percent THC strain can feel better than a 25 percent THC strain.

- The only real difference between different concentrates is personal preference. I find it easier to load shatter into my vaporizer while someone else prefers vaping wax. Choose the one you like, and try them all until you decide which one you like best.

- Vape pens are great to have around for emergencies like back pain and insomnia.

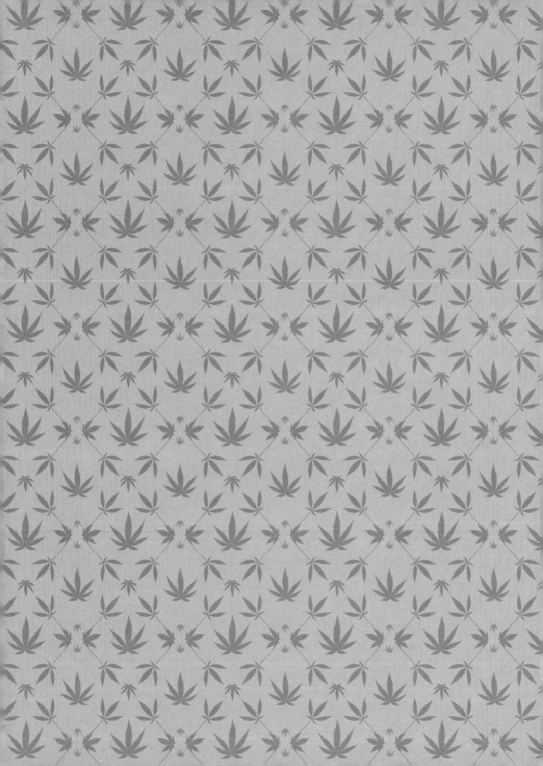

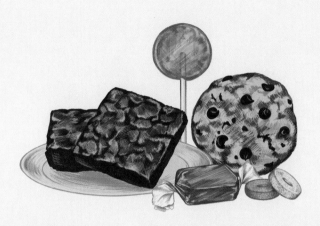

Part Five

EDIBLE CANNABIS—
CALM AND TASTY

Brownies, finally. You thought we were never going to get here, didn't you? Remember those concentrates we talked about in the last section? Even if you don't want to inhale them, you can use them to make your own edibles at home. If you skipped the inhaling section, but you want to make your own edibles, go back and read the section on cannabis concentrates (see page 124).

Even if you never plan to make your own edibles, understanding the process of making them will help you make better choices when you buy edibles at the dispensary.

INFUSIONS AND EXTRACTIONS

Since the dawn of time, people have infused marijuana into food and drink to use both as medicine and just for fun. Candy and chocolate, including gummies, brownies, and suckers, are the most popular edibles in dispensaries. There are dozens of other choices—nuts and dried fruit, granola, mints, coffee, sodas, teas, juices, cookies, popcorn, bacon, and ice cream.

The edibles available in your state are compliant with the laws in your state. Some states do not allow edibles that require refrigeration, so dispensaries cannot sell things like ice cream or lemon bars. Most states limit the THC in each edible, so if you need a higher dose, you have to buy more, which can get expensive.

When we make our own edibles at home, we save money, get the exact dose we want, and can use our favorite flavors and recipes. With a little math and a few tricks, every cookbook is a marijuana cookbook. Once you get comfortable with using cannabis extractions, you will be able to infuse cannabis into any recipe you like.

We can make any kind of brownie we want, but to get each brownie dosed with the same amount of THC, we need to follow a few guidelines.

- **PRACTICE THE RECIPE BEFORE INFUSING THE FOOD OR DRINK WITH CANNABIS.** Make a virgin batch with your own oven, molds, and measurements. When I first attempted toffee, I ruined the first four batches and lost more than $200 worth of cannabis.

- **STIR. STIR. STIR AGAIN.** Cannabis must be evenly distributed through the entire batch of dough, candy, or chocolate. Use silicone spatulas and heat to get marijuana properly distributed.

- **MAKE BITE-SIZED PORTIONS.** Think mini cupcakes, not a whole cake. Medicated cheese dip is fun, but do you really want to eat a whole bowl of it—or even a scoop every day? These are recipes that will give you a dose of marijuana in a bite-sized portion of food that can easily be incorporated into a healthy eating plan.

- **WHEN CUTTING BATCHES INTO PIECES, MAKE SURE EACH PORTION IS THE EXACT SAME SIZE,** otherwise the THC will vary wildly from piece to piece. Use molds, mini-muffin pans, rulers, and scales to make sure each piece is the exact same size as every other piece.

Marijuana edibles don't require special equipment beyond the basic tools in your kitchen, but I still like to use a separate set of baking sheets, Pyrex cups, strainers, spatulas, and bowls for marijuana. Cannabis will eventually stain everything with a greenish hue that is difficult to remove.

Tools for Accurately Dosed Edibles

- **COOKIE CUTTERS**—I use cookie cutters to make suckers, dog treats, gummies, and cookies.

- **DIGITAL SCALE**—Measuring ingredients by weight instead of volume makes it easier to get accurate, even doses.

- **MOLDS**—Find a cake and/or candy specialty store and be amazed at the variety of chocolate and hard-candy molds that are available. Most are just a few dollars and can be used over and over again, so if you plan to make edibles on a regular basis, stock up on molds and cookie cutters.

- **MUFFIN/CUPCAKE/BROWNIE TINS**—These are the perfect molds for baked goods.

- **MELON BALLER**—Makes accurately dosed scoops of anything.

- **8 X 8-INCH BAKING PAN AND RULER**—Use these to cut sizes precisely.

EDIBLE EXTRACTIONS

To turn a regular brownie into a "special" brownie, the cook first extracts THC and CBD from marijuana flowers. Then the extraction is infused into an edible like butter, oil, or alcohol. (Vanilla extract is created in basically the same way. The vanilla beans are infused into the alcohol.) Then the infused butter, oil, or alcohol is incorporated into foods, drinks, and skin treatments.

BUTTER—Fat is an excellent solvent for extracting medicinal compounds from marijuana, and the higher the fat content, the more potent the butter, which is why ghee, aka clarified butter, is most often used. Some dispensaries sell cannabutter, ready-infused for baking homemade edibles.

OILS—Olive oil and coconut oil strip more of the cannabinoids and terpenes from the plant matter than butter, which means that using oil will result in a more potent edible. Any oil can be used to extract cannabinoids and terpenes and used to make edibles and topicals for skin.

ALCOHOL—Soaking marijuana in a high-proof alcohol like Everclear will extract cannabinoids and terpenes into a highly potent, medicated liquid. Alcohol extractions can be used to make hard candy and other recipes without fat.

Cooking with Concentrates

Many commercial edible producers do not use cannabis flower to make their edibles. They use cannabis concentrates such as CO_2 oil to infuse food with marijuana, and so can we.

Making edibles from cannabis flower means the flower must be soaked and simmered in a solvent such as butter, oil, or alcohol before it is infused into food. It's a messy, time-consuming process.

Concentrates, on the other hand, have already been extracted from the flower, so they only need to be infused into food. When I buy a gram of CO_2 oil, it has around 700 milligrams of THC, the same amount I would get from 7 grams (a quarter) of cannabis flower. The gram of oil and quarter of flower cost about the same, and when I get home, I have one less step to do.

If your dispensary does not have CO_2 oil, choose another concentrate, such as wax or shatter. Just make sure that the concentrate is the THC:CBD ratio that you prefer. During the decarboxylation step, all concentrates will melt into a liquid, so it doesn't matter which concentrate you choose.

DECARBOXYLATION

"I ate an edible, but I didn't feel anything."

"These brownies were supposed to be super strong, but nothing happened."

When you cook with cannabis and don't feel the effects, the

most likely reason is that they were made with raw cannabis flower. Raw marijuana is not psychoactive—that is, it will not get us high. Marijuana plants contain THCA, the acid form of THC, and THCA is not psychoactive. When exposed to heat, like when smoking or vaping, THCA converts to THC and we get high.

Decarboxylation or *decarb* is the intimidating term for the process of heating marijuana until the THCA has converted to THC. This is the first step when creating any infused product. CBDA—the acid form of cannabinoids—is also present in the marijuana plant. It converts to CBD—the pain-relieving cannabinoid—when heated.

Concentrates are used to make infused edibles and topicals, and concentrates must be decarboxylated as well to convert THCA to THC. This usually happens when you smoke or vape it, but when you're cooking it, the heat of the oven infusing the edible does *not* work to covert the THCA to THC. It has to be done *before* you bake, since the heat of cooking the food is usually not hot enough to convert THCA to THC.

Different strains may need more time in the oven. THCA tends to convert more quickly to THC than CBDA converts to CBD. THC-heavy strains of flower might only need forty-five minutes, while high-CBD strains need an hour to fully convert the cannabinoids. Adjust the cooking time as needed to get the flowers bone dry and a nice warm brown color. If any bits of marijuana are still green, there is still THCA in the plant matter, which means it's not as potent as it could be. Return the flower to the oven until every bit has turned brown. At 250 degrees Fahrenheit, the flower won't burn, so don't worry about baking it too long.

For a lighter color and a more delicate flavor, blanch marijuana before decarboxylation. This process removes chlorophyll, which makes for a cleaner, lighter flavor. Just like blanching vegetables, drop marijuana into boiling water for three to four minutes, then quickly plunge into a bowl of ice water. Let dry, then grind and decarboxylate blanched marijuana flowers.

After the flower has been heated, spraying it with alcohol like Everclear will break down the cellulose, which reduces the green hue of the infused butter, oil, or alcohol. Decarboxylation releases moisture, which results in a 10 to 12 percent decrease in weight, so an ounce of marijuana (28 grams) dries out to 24 to 25 grams. Decarboxylation causes a heavy scent, so turn on the vent, open the windows, and position fans to blow the scent to the great outdoors.

DECARBOXYLATION, STEP-BY-STEP

Yield: 24 to 25 grams of decarboxylated marijuana

INGREDIENTS

Ice

Cannabis flower

Everclear (if you cannot buy
high-proof alcohol in your state,
use vodka)

EQUIPMENT

Heavy pot

Bowl

Slotted spoon

Fine-mesh wire rack or cardboard

Grinder

Baking sheet

Foil

Small spray bottle

Airtight jar

1. Preheat the oven to 250°F.

2. In a heavy pot, bring a few cups of water to a boil. In a bowl, make an ice bath.

3. Add the cannabis flower to the boiling water for 3 to 4 minutes, then remove it from the boiling water with a slotted spoon and transfer it to the ice bath to cool for 1 minute. Remove the flower from the ice bath and lay it out on cardboard or a fine-mesh wire rack to dry about 30 minutes.

4. Coarsely grind the flower into the texture of tobacco. Place the ground flower on a baking sheet in a thin layer. Cover the baking sheet with foil.

5. Bake for 30 minutes. Pull from the oven, then shake the tray to stir. Return to the oven for another 30 minutes. When ready, the flower will be a lightly toasted brown color, not green.

6. Remove from the oven, keep covered, and allow to cool for 15 minutes. Remove foil.

7. Spray cannabis with a light coating of Everclear (or vodka) to break down cellulose. This step will reduce any potential green hue of the butter, oil, or alcohol infusion. Allow the flower to dry for about 20 minutes.

8. When dry, store the flower in an airtight jar in a cool, dry place. Decarboxylated flower can be stored for a few months or used immediately.

Butter Extractions

Now that the cannabis is decarboxylated, the next step is to extract the medicinally beneficial cannabinoids and terpenes from the flowers and infuse them into a solvent like butter or oil.

Butter is a wonderful solvent to extract cannabinoids and terpenes. A lovely jar of medicated butter can be used for any kind of edible. When I get vegetables that I don't love in my CSA share, I douse them in butter and salt and roast them, and suddenly I'm eating brussels sprouts like candy. Sweets like brownies and cookies and caramels become delicious medicine. Add a teaspoon to coffee or a piece of toast for a medicated morning.

I can't tell if butter from grass-fed, self-actualized cows really tastes better, but Michael Pollan convinced me it is true, so sometimes I spend a few extra dollars on the good stuff. Regular sticks of unsalted butter also work just fine—but definitely stay away from margarine and fake butters. We want butterfat, not chemicals, because fat is what extracts cannabinoids and terpenes from the plant matter.

Simmering the butter for a few minutes before adding marijuana makes a more potent butter. Elaine Khosrova, author of *Butter: A Rich History*, taught me that all ghee is clarified butter, but not all clarified butter is ghee. Clarified butter extracts more cannabinoids and terpenes than regular butter because clarified butter has more butterfat and less water. Ghee will extract even more because it has less water and more butterfat as a result of being cooked longer. Browned butter has less water, like ghee, and also has a flavorful taste that helps cover the flavor of marijuana.

CLARIFIED BUTTER/GHEE/BROWNED BUTTER

Yield: 1 pound of clarified butter, ghee, or browned butter

INGREDIENTS

1 pound plus ¼ cup unsalted
   butter

EQUIPMENT

Medium-sized saucepan,
   preferably with heavy bottom
Spoon
Coffee filter
Fine-mesh strainer
mason jar

1. In a medium-sized saucepan, melt the butter over medium-low heat for 5 to 10 minutes. The butter will separate into layers, with foam developing on top and milk solids sinking to the bottom. Keep an eye on the heat to prevent burning the milk solids. The simmer should barely move the surface of the butter, with a few bubbles appearing to release water.

2. After about 15 minutes, use a spoon to skim and discard the top layer of foam. Keep an eye on the color of the milk solids at the bottom.

3. For clarified butter, remove the pot from the heat when the milk solids turn a light-brown color.

4. For ghee, keep the pan on the heat until the milk solids turn a toasted-brown color. When they do, strain the butter through a coffee filter in a fine-mesh strainer to separate the solids from the now-clarified butter. Discard the solids or save for another use.

5. For browned butter, continue to cook to a deep golden brown but *don't* strain out the milk solids after they are cooked. Browned butter is a blink away from burned butter, so keep an eye on the heat and the milk solids as they finish cooking. Remove the butter from the heat and pour it into a mason jar.

6. Cool. For all three butters, store in a mason jar in the fridge for several weeks.

CANNABUTTER TIPS

- If you want homemade cannabutter more easily, try using a butter-making machine. Much like a bread machine, you simply add ingredients and press start. Try the MagicalButter machine.

- You can also purchase clarified butter and ghee at the grocery store to skip that step, too.

- *Bioavailability* refers to how effectively the body will absorb and utilize the medicinal cannabinoids and terpenes. To increase the bioavailability of THC and CBD, add 2 to 3 tablespoons of liquid lecithin for every stick of butter. Lecithin increases the number of milligrams of THC/CBD that the body absorbs, which means 10 milligrams with lecithin gets us higher than 10 milligrams without it. Lecithin is an emulsifier, which means it makes oil and water bind together instead of separate. Chocolate has lecithin to maintain the emulsion of cocoa butter, sugar, and cocoa paste. I like to use liquid soy lecithin (granulated lecithin is clumpy), but there is sunflower, soy, or egg yolk lecithin, and they come in liquid and granulated forms. Do not use any lecithin in caramel or toffee recipes. The extra emulsion prevents the sugar from caramelizing properly.

- Invest in a fine-mesh strainer. Cannabis plant matter needs to be filtered from butters, oils, and alcohol after the extraction process. Straining can be messy, and I've found that a fine-mesh strainer is tidier than cheesecloth. Press hard to get every drop of medicated butter from the cannabis, and throw out the plant matter when you're finished straining.

- The flavor of cannabutter depends on the quality and flavor of both the marijuana and butter that go into it. If the plant matter is mostly flower with a thick coating of trichomes, the butter will be strongly scented and flavored. If less marijuana flavor is desired, choose flower that has fewer terpenes, but remember that reducing terpenes reduces the effectiveness of the medicine as well as the flavor.

- If your cannabutter has a very strong cannabis flavor, you can tone it down by adding other flavors, what we call compound butter. Stir in a few tablespoons of honey for infused honey butter. I like to add a teaspoon of vanilla extract and a dash of nutmeg. In the summer, add herbs from the garden.

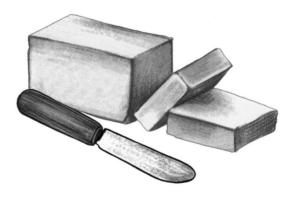

FLOWER CANNABUTTER

Yield: ½ cup of flower cannabutter

INGREDIENTS

½ cup plus 2 tablespoons unsalted
    butter
3.5 grams (for a mild effect) or
    7 grams (for a strong effect)
    decarboxylated cannabis flower
2 tablespoons liquid lecithin

EQUIPMENT

Medium-sized pot or saucepan
Small jar or glass measuring cup
Whisk
Fine-mesh strainer or cheesecloth
Airtight jar

1. Fill a medium-sized pot or saucepan halfway with water and set to boil.

2. In a small jar or glass measuring cup, combine the butter with the cannabis flower. Set the uncovered jar in boiling water. When the butter has melted, whisk the mixture to evenly coat the cannabis.

3. Reduce the heat and simmer the mixture for 1 hour. Add more water as needed.

4. Allow the mixture to cool, then strain it through a fine-mesh strainer or cheesecloth. Firmly press to squeeze out every single drop of medicated butter. Strain again. It will result in ½ cup of butter.

5. Add the lecithin and stir well until blended.

6. Store the cannabutter in an airtight jar in the fridge for up to a month or freeze for up to 6 months.

CANNABUTTER MATH

The best thing about dispensary edibles is that the label tells us exactly how many milligrams of THC and CBD are in each edible. But when we make them at home, we have to figure out the potency in each treat. If we have the potency test results for the flower, it's just a few quick steps to figure out the number of milligrams per edible.

STEP 1: Check the package label for your flower. Add together the THC and THCA potency for the total THC potency (aka the percentage of THC in the flower). Add CBD and CBDA for the total CBD potency. Remember that THCA converts to THC when heated; that is why we need to add them together to get the total percent of THC.

STEP 2: Convert potency percentages to milligrams. This sounds more complicated than it is. Each gram of cannabis flower is 1,000 milligrams. If THC is 20 percent, that means 200 of the 1,000 total milligrams are THC.

5 percent THC = 50 milligrams
10 percent THC = 100 milligrams
15 percent THC = 150 milligrams
20 percent THC = 200 milligrams

STEP 3: Divide this number in half. Unfortunately, not all of the THC in the flower is going to end up in the butter. Some THC is lost during the decarboxylation process, and some is lost during the extraction process. As a general rule of thumb, we assume that half of the THC/CBD is lost, so we divide the total number of milligrams by two.

STEP 4: Multiply the number of milligrams in 1 gram by the number of grams of flower you are using. If your flower is 100 milligrams THC per gram, and you have 7 grams of it, you have 700 milligrams.

STEP 5: Divide the total number of milligrams by the number of servings in the batch, and you have the number of milligrams in each piece. So if you make 20 brownies with your 700 milligrams, each brownie has 35 milligrams.

In the recipes made with cannabutter, it is always ½ cup in an 8 x 8-inch baking pan, and it is divided into either 16 or 32 servings. For mild doses and a mild high, use less cannabis and cut more pieces. For a stronger dose and a stronger high, use more cannabis and cut the batch into fewer pieces.

How to make 32 brownies with 20 milligrams THC each:
7 grams flower = 20 percent THC/CBD potency
8 x 8-inch baking pan
Cut into 1 x 2-inch pieces

How to make 64 brownies with 5 milligrams THC each:
3.5 grams flower = 20 percent THC/CBD potency
8 x 8-inch baking pan
Cut into 1 x 1-inch pieces

Flower, Trim, and Shake in Your Butter

In the dispensary, cannabis is sold by the gram, usually in 3.5- or 7-gram containers. If you use 3.5 grams of a high-THC flower and infuse it into a half cup (one stick) of butter, you'll end up with about 350 to 450 milligrams of THC in the butter. If you use 7 grams of a high-THC flower, you'll have around 700 to 800 milligrams of THC in your half cup of butter.

We can also use cannabis trim or shake instead of flower. *Trim* refers to the sugar leaves and tiny flower buds from the bottom of the plant. We don't smoke trim, but we can use it to cook. *Shake* is cannabis flower than has been broken down and is no longer in a bud shape. When we grind up flower to smoke it, we are making shake.

Shake and trim tend to be less expensive at the dispensary, but they are also less potent, so to get stronger doses, we need to use more shake or trim.

CANNABUTTER MATH AT A GLANCE		
TO INFUSE ½ CUP BUTTER...	FOR A MILD DOSE OF 250–500 MILLIGRAMS...	FOR A STRONG DOSE OF 500–800 MILLIGRAMS...
Using trim or shake...	You need 7 grams.	You need 14 grams.
Using flower...	You need 3.5 grams.	You need 7 grams.
Using concentrate...	You need ½ gram.	You need 1 gram.

Cannabis-Infused Oils

When infusing cannabis into food and skin treatments, oils are more versatile than butter. Olive, coconut, grapeseed, peanut, canola, and other oils can be used to make both sweet and savory edibles even better. Salad dressing, kale chips, bacon, cakes, and even mayonnaise can be infused with marijuana. Boxed cake, brownie, and muffin mixes all use oil rather than butter for a super-moist crumb. This does not extend to frying, though, as medicinal compounds will be destroyed before an oil gets hot enough to fry foods.

Tinctures are infused alcohol that delivers a concentrated dose. But many find that fractionated coconut oil is a tastier and healthier choice for making tinctures. Fractionated coconut oil is a pure liquid at room temperature and does not smell or taste like coconuts. It differs from virgin coconut oil, which stays solid at room temperature and has a distinct coconut smell and flavor. Both forms of coconut oil make great-tasting edibles.

Cannabis-infused oils make luxurious antiaging topical creams and lotions that moisturize skin and relieve pain. When used in a topical application, fractionated coconut oil penetrates the skin quickly and doesn't feel greasy. Topicals made from solid coconut oil feel greasier on the skin and tend to cause breakouts, but are more beneficial for infections and conditions like eczema and psoriasis.

Oil doesn't evaporate like butter or alcohol, and oil extracts more cannabinoids from cannabis than butter.

FLOWER OIL EXTRACTION

Yield: 1 ounce cannabis-infused oil

INGREDIENTS

1½ ounces oil
3.5 grams (for a mild effect)
   or 7 grams (strong effect)
   decarboxylated cannabis flower

EQUIPMENT

Medium-sized pot or saucepan
Small jar or glass measuring cup
Fine-mesh strainer or cheesecloth
1-ounce bottle with dropper top

1. Fill a medium-sized pot or saucepan halfway with water and set to boil.

2. In a small jar or glass measuring cup, combine the oil and cannabis. Set the container in boiling water.

3. Simmer for 1 hour.

4. Allow the mixture to cool, then strain it through a fine-mesh strainer or cheesecloth. Firmly press to squeeze out every single drop of medicated oil. Strain again.

5. Store the extraction in a 1-ounce bottle with a dropper top in a cool, dry place for up to 6 months.

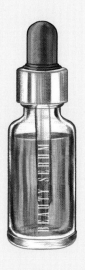

CANNAOIL TIPS

- Oil doesn't evaporate, so we can't reduce it like an alcohol tincture. If you want a single ounce of very potent oil, use the highest-potency flower you can find. (Do not use shake or trim. An ounce of oil simply can't absorb 14 grams of trim.)

- For very potent cannaoil, use a gram of cannabis concentrate like wax or shatter. Simply decarboxylate the concentrate in the oven for 30 minutes at 250 degrees Fahrenheit. During the last minute, microwave, on high heat, an ounce of oil. When both are hot, blend the concentrate with the oil.

- Just like an alcohol tincture, apply a cannabis-infused oil tincture under the tongue for a sublingual application that skips the digestive system and provides pain relief and mood elevation faster.

- To create cannaoil that provides pain relief without the high, use a low-THC, high-CBD strain, or use a high-THC strain and skip the decarboxylation step. If you don't bake the cannabis before you infuse it into the oil, you've made an oil that reduces pain and inflammation without a high. This is ideal for pets and children, too.

Alcohol Extractions

Before 1937, apothecaries stocked marijuana tinctures to cure everything that ailed us. Before pharmaceutical sales reps and the FDA, doctors and pharmacists mixed marijuana concoctions to relieve pain and improve sleep. Before we get too nostalgic for the good old days, let's also remember that our recent ancestors had leeches applied to their skin medicinally, no penicillin, and a much shorter life span.

A sublingual application is when the body absorbs the medicine through the soft tissues of the mouth instead of traveling through the digestive system. Placing drops of tincture under the tongue gets cannabinoids to the endocannabinoid system much faster, which means the medicinal effects of the marijuana take effect sooner than by digesting marijuana in an edible. Sublingual applications skip the journey through the stomach and liver, which strips away some of the cannabinoids and reduces the bioavailability of cannabinoids that are absorbed into the bloodstream.

Alcohol extractions are more potent when they are made from the highest proof alcohol available. Everclear is the standard against which all other alcohols are measured. It is 190 proof, which means it is almost pure alcohol. Vodka, bourbon, and other hard liquors are only 80 proof, which means they are less than 50 percent alcohol. I also like to use moonshine or absinthe for my alcohol solvent, but Everclear extracts more of the cannabinoids and terpenes from the plant matter. Check with your local liquor store to see if they stock Everclear, because it is a bit harder to find than other alcohols. Some states have banned the sale of 190 proof Everclear. If 190 proof alcohol is not available in your area, look for 151 proof.

Tinctures can be made without heat and without odor, simply by placing decarboxylated marijuana in a jar, pouring enough alcohol over it to fully immerse the plant matter, and screwing on an airtight lid. Give the jar a shake and place it in a cool, dark place for a few weeks. Then, strain the plant matter out of the liquid and toss the plant matter. The strained alcohol is now a thin, green liquid, ready to get us high and happy. Add flavorings like vanilla beans, citrus rinds, peppermint, rosemary, ginger, or chamomile. Tinctures don't need to be refrigerated, and they last for several months.

The difference between a fat extraction and an alcohol extraction is that alcohol evaporates and fat does not. If you simmer a cup of olive oil for hours, you'll still have a cup of olive oil. Alcohol evaporates too quickly to simmer for hours. Once, I wandered away from the stove during an alcohol extraction and all the liquid evaporated until I had nothing but ruined plant matter and a burned jar. When making an extraction with alcohol, you always want to use lower heat and less of a boil than a butter or oil extraction.

Evaporation works in our favor because it allows us to make a liquid so potent that just a few drops will get us high or relieve our pain. If you finish your tincture and decide that it isn't strong enough, put it back on a low heat and reduce it, like cooking down a sauce.

Tincture can also be made with vegetable glycerin, using the exact same process. Glycerin does not extract as many cannabinoids and terpenes as alcohol, so the final product will not be as potent. However, glycerin is alcohol-free and tastes much, much better than alcohol, so if you are making tincture for a child, use glycerin.

Do not try to make an unheated alcohol extraction with a concentrate like wax or shatter. They simply don't melt into alcohol without heat.

CANNABIS TINCTURE

Alcohol is flammable, so be careful near heat. It also evaporates quickly, so if you plan to simmer longer, add more Everclear (or vodka).

Yield: 1 ounce of flower tincture

INGREDIENTS
2 ounces Everclear (or vodka)
3.5 grams (for a mild effect) or
   7 grams (for a strong effect)
   decarboxylated cannabis flower

EQUIPMENT
Medium-sized pot or saucepan
Small jar or glass measuring cup
Whisk
Fine-mesh strainer or cheesecloth
1-ounce bottle with dropper top

1. In a medium-sized pot or saucepan, boil 2 to 3 cups water.

2. Put the alcohol into a small jar or glass measuring cup. Whisk in the cannabis flower. Set the container in the boiling water.

3. Simmer for 30 to 45 minutes.

4. Allow the mixture to cool, then strain it through the a fine-mesh strainer or cheesecloth. Firmly press to squeeze out every single drop of tincture. Strain again.

5. Store the tincture in 1-ounce bottle with a dropper top in a cool, dry place for up to 6 months.

TINCTURE MATH

To find the amount of THC and CBD in each dose of edibles made with tincture, we use the same math we used for cannabutter and cannabis oil.

STEP 1: Add THC and THCA for the total THC potency. Add CBD and CBDA for the total CBD potency. Remember that THCA coverts to THC, so we need to add them together to get the total amount of THC.

STEP 2: Convert the percentage to milligrams. This sounds more complicated than it is. Each gram of cannabis flower is 1,000 milligrams. If THC is 20 percent, that means 200 of those milligrams are THC.

5 percent THC = 50 milligrams
10 percent THC = 100 milligrams
15 percent THC = 150 milligrams
20 percent THC = 200 milligrams

STEP 3: Divide this number in half. Unfortunately, not all of the THC in the flower is going to end up in the tincture. Some THC is lost during the decarboxylation process and some is lost during the extraction process. As a rule of thumb, we assume that half of the THC/CBD is lost, so we divide the total number of milligrams by two.

STEP 4: Multiply the number of milligrams in 1 gram by the number of grams of flower you are using. If your flower is 100 milligrams

THC per gram of flower and you have 7 grams of it, you have 700 milligrams.

STEP 5: Divide the total number of milligrams by the number of servings in the batch, and you have the number of milligrams in each piece. So if you make 20 suckers with your 700 milligrams, each sucker has 35 milligrams.

TINCTURE TIPS

• After you finish the process and your tincture is strained, leave it out overnight, uncovered, on the kitchen counter. Some of the alcohol will evaporate and the remaining liquid will be more potent. Let it sit out to evaporate until you have the amount of liquid you want, then store it in an airtight container.

• Tincture is stored in blue or amber glass bottles with dropper tops. A one-ounce bottle holds thirty doses and a half-ounce bottle holds fifteen doses. (Each dose is the amount the dropper top sucks up out of the bottle.)

• Tincture doesn't taste good, and the alcohol can feel like a burn on the tongue, so squirt the tincture under your tongue to avoid tasting it.

• Because tincture soaks into the soft tissues of the mouth, it is called a sublingual application. This means the THC is stronger and kicks in faster than with an edible—which loses some of its potency to the liver.

EDIBLE RECIPES

HYSTERICAL-FIT TRUFFLES

Alice B. Toklas included a recipe for hashish fudge in her 1954 cookbook, *The Alice B. Toklas Cook Book*. She called it "the food of paradise" and said two pieces would produce hysterical fits of laughter and "wild floods of thought on many simultaneous planes." I promise you, Alice had more than 10 milligrams of THC in each piece. Ten milligrams of THC will not send you to simultaneous planes. But it will reduce your risk of dementia and boost your mood.

While Alice called her recipe "fudge," it was really more like the following nutritional powerhouse. Walnuts, almonds, and cashews blend well into a paste, and prunes hold the mixture together. Other nuts, seeds, or dried fruits can be added. Coat truffles in anything from toasted sesame seeds to chocolate nibs.

Yield: 15 (strong) or 30 (mild) truffles

Infusion: Use cannabis flower infused in coconut oil (see page 153 for recipe). Do not use marijuana concentrate directly. Without heat, the concentrate won't melt and blend into the mixture.

Strain: Choose a high-THC sativa strain for maximum hysterical fits.

INGREDIENTS

3.5 grams (for a mild effect) or 7 grams (for a strong effect) cannabis flower

1½ ounces coconut oil

1½ cups chopped walnuts, almonds, or cashews

1 cup pitted prunes

1 tablespoon vanilla extract

½ cup chopped dried cherries

½ cup crushed and toasted pistachio nuts

EQUIPMENT

Food processor or blender

Airtight container

1. Infuse cannabis flower into coconut oil (see page 153 for recipe).

2. Add the cannabis-infused coconut oil, walnuts, prunes, and vanilla extract to the food processor or blender. Blend into a sticky paste.

3. Stir in the chopped cherries.

4. Roll the paste into 15 to 30 balls.

5. Roll each ball through a shallow dish of crushed pistachio nuts until evenly coated.

6. Store refrigerated in an airtight container for 2 to 3 weeks.

CLASSIC POT BROWNIES

Lately, my daily uniform is a black dress and ballet flats. I'm not Steve Jobs about it—I have dresses in varying lengths, silhouettes, and fabrics, but this uniform keeps my life, my closet, and my laundry simple and easy. These brownies are like black dresses and ballet flats. Fast and simple but perfect and delicious.

Chocolate has medicinal compounds that make us almost as happy and healthy as cannabis. In fact, chocolate already contains small amounts of cannabinoids. Cacao beans are loaded with antioxidants, magnesium, and serotonin and other feel-good compounds, which makes chocolate edibles so popular at the dispensary and the most delicious and effective edibles we can make at home.

The rich flavor covers the cannabis taste well, but for more chocolate richness, add a tablespoon of cocoa powder. Sometimes I add a few cranks of black pepper or a dash or two of nutmeg, cinnamon, or cardamom, just for fun.

Yield: 16 (strong) or 32 (mild) brownies

Infusion: Use cannabis-flower-infused butter (see page 148 for recipe).

Strain: Choose a medium-potency hybrid THC strain for a classic high.

INGREDIENTS

3.5 grams (for a mild effect) or
    7 grams (for a strong effect)
    cannabis flower
½ cup plus 2 tablespoons butter
3 ounces unsweetened chocolate
Nonstick cooking spray
1⅓ cups sugar
2 large eggs
2 teaspoons vanilla extract
½ teaspoon salt

⅔ cup flour
Flaky sea salt

EQUIPMENT

Small heatproof bowl
Whisk
8 x 8-inch baking pan
Ruler
Toothpicks
Plastic or parchment paper

1. Infuse cannabis flower into butter (see page 148 for recipe). The result will be a ½ cup of cannabis butter. Soften before using.

2. Preheat oven to 350°F. Spray nonstick cooking spray or line an 8 x 8-inch baking pan with parchment paper.

3. In a small heatproof bowl, microwave the chocolate in 30-second bursts until melted. Add the softened cannabutter and stir well. All the stirring is best done by hand.

4. Add the sugar and stir. Beat in the eggs one at a time. Stir in the vanilla and salt. Add the flour and gently stir until the batter is smooth.

5. Pour the batter into an 8 x 8-inch baking pan and sprinkle with flaky sea salt.

6. Bake for 25 to 30 minutes, until a crust forms on top and a toothpick comes out clean.

7. Cool the brownies and cut them into thirty-two 1 x 1-inch pieces or sixteen 2 x 2-inch pieces. Use a ruler to make even cuts.

8. Cover and store the brownies at room temperature for a week or individually wrap in plastic or parchment paper to freeze up to 6 months.

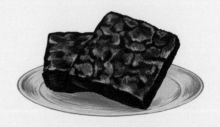

Hard Candy

Hard candies are a sweet, discreet way of medicating on the go, and they can be made in any dose, color, flavor, size, or shape. Understanding hard-crack temperatures and pouring syrup quickly before it solidifies seem intimidating at first, but once you get the hang of it, you'll be making professional-looking, gourmet marijuana candies in your own kitchen.

Hard crack is the hottest stage of candy making, and the temperature is a precise 300 degrees Fahrenheit. If the syrup does not get heated to 300 degrees, the candy will be sticky and soft. If the syrup is cooked over 305 degrees, it will caramelize and turn brown. Heat the sugar syrup on a high heat. Longer cook times increase browning of the syrup. Heating the solution as quickly as possible keeps the color clear and prevents caramelization of the syrup.

Add food coloring one drop at a time. For pretty sea glass, I make two batches—one blue and one green—and then mix them. Sometimes I do a light blue and a dark blue, and the difference is only a drop or two.

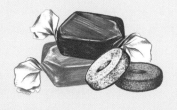

Basic flavoring is available in specialty food shops and online. Without flavoring, the cannabis taste will be noticeable.

Do not attempt hard candy without a candy thermometer. Trust me.

BARELY HIGH SEA GLASS

Yield: 16 (strong) or 32 (mild) quarter-ounce servings

Infusion: Use cannabis infused in alcohol (see page 157 for recipe).

Strain: Choose a low-THC, high-CBD hybrid strain for a powerful dose of pain relief without a high.

INGREDIENTS

3.5 grams (for a mild effect) or 7 grams (for a strong effect) cannabis flower

2 ounces Everclear (or vodka)

Nonstick cooking spray

1 cup granulated sugar

¼ cup water

¼ cup light corn syrup

2–3 drops food coloring

1 teaspoon flavoring

1 cup powdered sugar

EQUIPMENT

8 x 8-inch baking pan

Heavy pot

Small brush

Candy thermometer

Silicone spatula

Pyrex measuring cup

Food scale

1. Infuse cannabis into Everclear (or vodka) (see page 157 for recipe).

2. Spray an 8 x 8-inch baking pan with nonstick cooking spray.

3. In a heavy pot, mix the sugar and water over high heat. Stir until all of the sugar dissolves. Use a small brush to wipe the mixture from the sides of the pot.

4. Add the corn syrup and food coloring. Attach a candy thermometer to the pot and bring the mixture to a boil. Do not stir as the temperature rises. Prepare an ice bath large enough to hold the pot.

5. At 300°F, remove pot from heat and place in an ice bath.

6. When the syrup has stopped boiling, add flavoring and infused alcohol. Use a small silicone spatula and stir well.

7. Pour the syrup into the baking pan. Tilt the pan back and forth to evenly spread syrup. Allow to cool at room temperature.

8. When set, break the sheet into bite-sized pieces.

9. Lightly coat each piece with powdered sugar to keep them from sticking together. Use a food scale to measure out quarter-ounce servings. Store in a cool, dry place for a few weeks.

Caramel

Caramel is sugar, dairy, and fat, the perfect combination for marijuana medicine. The fat and dairy help our bodies absorb more of the marijuana, and the sugar makes it taste good.

For different flavors, substitute coconut cream for cow's milk cream, or use honey, maple syrup, or agave instead of white sugar and corn syrup. Dried lavender is a lovely addition. So is booze. A quarter cup of bourbon added to the sugar mixture adds a unique flavor, and if you really want to get crazy, use eggnog instead of cream.

Making great caramel requires a candy thermometer, and cutting caramels into evenly sized pieces requires a pizza cutter.

NETFLIX AND CHILL CARAMELS

The danger with these caramels is that they are so delicious you may keep eating them and get way too high. Think about making a virgin batch of caramel to snack on during your Netflix binge. Label correctly!

Yield: 16 (strong) or 32 (mild) caramels

Infusion: Use cannabis flower infused into butter (see page 148 for recipe). Do not use lecithin in the cannabutter because the extra emulsion prevents the caramel from setting up properly.

Strain: Choose a high-THC strain from the indica section of the dispensary. Look for myrcene and linalool terpenes for maximum relaxation.

INGREDIENTS

3.5 grams (for a mild effect) or
7 grams (for a strong effect)
cannabis flower

½ cup (4 ounces, 1 stick) unsalted
butter, clarified butter, or ghee

½ cup water

1 cup granulated sugar

¼ cup light corn syrup

½ cup heavy cream
(at least 36% butterfat)

1 tablespoon vanilla extract

1 teaspoon salt

Optional: flaky sea salt

EQUIPMENT

8 x 8-inch baking pan or
candy molds

Parchment paper or nonstick
cooking spray

Medium-sized saucepan

Candy thermometer

Whisk

Silicone spatula

Pizza cutter

Airtight container

1. Infuse cannabis into butter (see page 148 for recipe).

2. Line an 8 x 8-inch baking pan with parchment paper or spray pan or molds with nonstick cooking spray.

3. In a medium-sized saucepan, bring the water, sugar, and corn syrup to a boil. Using a candy thermometer, cook until the sugar reaches 270°F. Remove from heat.

4. Slowly add the cream and cannabutter using a whisk. Mixture will double in size. Return the pan to a medium heat. Stirring constantly, allow the mixture to rise to 240–250°F. It will take 5 to 10 minutes. Remove from heat.

5. Add the vanilla extract and salt. Stir well until blended.

6. Carefully pour the mixture into the 8 x 8-inch baking pan or molds.

7. Optional: Sprinkle flaky sea salt over the caramel. Let the mixture cool to room temperature for at least an hour.

8. If you used a pan rather than molds, cut the caramel into pieces with a pizza cutter. Wrap each piece in parchment paper and store them in an airtight container in a cool, dry place for several months.

Gummy Candy

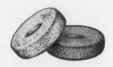

Gummies are one of the most popular products in dispensaries, and they are a popular recipe to make at home, too. Gummies have a long shelf life and can be made with healthy, tasty ingredients. We get to play with colors and flavors like hard candy, but gummy syrup gives us more time to work before the syrup sets, unlike the quick-setting sugar syrup for hard candy. Honey or maple syrup can be used instead of sugar, and grass-fed gelatin is all the rage with the paleo crowd. Extra packets of gelatin will make the candy gummier. Both pectin and gelatin are gelling agents and either can be used for gummies or *pâte de fruits*. Gelatin is not vegan, but pectin is a plant-based thickener. Gelatin needs to bloom, but it is easier to work with than pectin. Gelatin uses any liquid to work its magic. Pectin requires a lot of sugar (don't use honey with pectin) and acidity to set up properly.

BOOK CLUB WINE GUMMIES

I advise you NOT to mix marijuana with alcohol. You will probably get sick.

That said, there is one way to do it—in a gummy. Mixing THC with a dash of wine is a relaxing good time. Each piece has a tablespoon of wine, so it's a communion wine serving, not a happy hour serving. Wine gummies are more for wine flavor than intoxication, so choose your favorite red, white, or rosé.

Yield: 16 (strong) or 32 (mild) gummies. If using molds, don't use a shape that's appealing to a child. Stick with small basic shapes for safety.

Infusion: Use cannabis flower infused into an alcohol tincture (see page 157 for recipe).

Strain: For a great discussion, choose a happy sativa THC strain.

INGREDIENTS

3.5 grams (for a mild effect) or
   7 grams (for a strong effect)
   cannabis flower
1½ ounces Everclear (or vodka)
4 packets unflavored gelatin
1 cup red, white, or rosé wine,
   divided into 2 half cups
½ cup sugar

EQUIPMENT

8 x 8-inch baking dish or
   candy molds
Parchment paper or nonstick
   cooking spray
Bowl
Saucepan
Silicone spatula
Ruler
Pizza cutter
Wire rack
Airtight container

1. Infuse cannabis into Everclear (or vodka) (see page 157 for recipe).

2. Line an 8 x 8-inch baking dish with parchment paper or spray molds with nonstick cooking spray.

3. In a bowl, combine the 4 packets of gelatin with one of the two half cups of wine. Stir. Let the mixture sit for 5 to 10 minutes to allow the gelatin to absorb the liquid.

4. In a small saucepan, combine the sugar with the second half cup of wine. Bring the mixture to a boil and simmer it for 5 to 10 minutes, until thickened to a syrup consistency.

5. Add the gelatin mixture to the sugar syrup and stir until it is all melted together into a liquid. Add the cannabis tincture. Stir well.

6. Remove the mixture from the heat. Pour it into an 8 x 8-inch baking dish and refrigerate for 20 minutes until the gummies have set.

7. Remove the gummies mixture from the dish and cut it into evenly sized pieces with a ruler and pizza cutter. Set them out on a wire rack for a few hours to dry. Store them in an airtight container in the fridge for up to 2 weeks. Freezing them will change the texture and isn't recommended.

SUNDAY BRUNCH STRAWBERRY BALSAMIC *PÂTE DE FRUITS*

Pâte de fruits are grown-up gummies, flavored with real fruit and rolled in sugar. It's like biting into the soul of a fruit. We can make these chewy bites with literally any fruit, so grab whatever is in season.

The strong fruity flavor and sweetness of fruit pâte do a good job of covering up the flavor of marijuana. For a flavor that matches your cannabis, use mango or pineapple puree seasoned with cloves and black pepper.

Yield: 16 (strong) or 32 (mild) doses

Infusion: Use cannabis infused in alcohol (see page 157 for recipe).

Strain: Choose a high-potency 1:1 THC/CBD sativa to feel high, social, and pain-free during downtime.

INGREDIENTS

3.5 grams (for a mild effect) or 7 grams (for a strong effect) cannabis flower

1½ ounces Everclear (or vodka)

1 pound fresh or frozen strawberries, defrosted, stemmed, and hulled

2 tablespoons balsamic vinegar

1 tablespoon dry pectin

1 cup granulated sugar

⅓ cup light corn syrup

2 teaspoons lemon juice

Granulated sugar for dusting

EQUIPMENT

8 x 8-inch baking dish or candy molds

Plastic wrap or nonstick cooking spray

Blender

Heavy pot

Whisk

Bowl

Candy thermometer

Silicone spatula

Ruler

Pizza cutter

Wire rack or parchment paper

Airtight container

Optional: paper candy cups

1. Infuse cannabis into Everclear (or vodka) (see page 157 for recipe).

2. Line an 8 x 8-inch baking dish with plastic wrap (not parchment paper or foil), or spray molds with nonstick cooking spray.

3. In a blender, puree the strawberries until they are smooth.

4. In a heavy pot, combine the strawberries and balsamic vinegar. Bring the mixture to a boil, stirring constantly.

5. Whisk together the pectin and sugar in a separate bowl and add the mixture to the puree, stirring. Add the light corn syrup and, using a candy thermometer, bring the temperature up to 225°F with a medium heat. Stir constantly with silicone spatula. This may take up to 5 minutes. Remove from heat and add the lemon juice and cannabis tincture.

6. Pour the mixture into the baking dish and let it sit for several hours at room temperature, or refrigerate it for faster setting. When set, remove the mixture from the dish by lifting up the plastic wrap. Cut it into evenly sized pieces with a ruler and a pizza cutter.

7. Dry the pieces overnight, covered, on a wire rack or on parchment paper. Toss them gently in granulated sugar. Store them for several weeks in an airtight container with parchment paper separating the layers, or use those cute little paper candy cups to look fancy.

WAKE 'N' BACON

Friends drop everything and come over when I make this bacon. Sometimes I save some for my dog as an extra-special treat. Crumble the bacon into bits and sprinkle it over chocolate ice cream or a salad. Use crumbled bacon as a coating for truffles or stir bits into chocolate-bacon bars. I have made chocolate bars with whole pieces of bacon in them. They have never lasted more than a day in my house, but they should be delicious for up to a week.

Yield: 16 (strong) half-slice or 32 (mild) quarter-slice servings

Infusion: Use a cannabis-infused alcohol tincture
(see page 157 for the recipe).

Strain: Use a 1:1 THC/CBD sativa for pain-free mornings.

INGREDIENTS
3.5 grams (for a mild effect) or
   7 grams (for a strong effect)
   cannabis flower
1½ ounce Everclear (or vodka)
8 strips thick-cut bacon
2 tablespoons brown sugar
1 tablespoon Dijon mustard

EQUIPMENT
2 baking sheets
Small bowl
Spoon
Wire rack or paper towels
Airtight container

1. Infuse cannabis flower into Everclear (or vodka) (see page 157 for recipe).

2. Preheat the oven to 375°F.

3. Lay the bacon on a baking sheet that has sides to catch any drips. Bake for 20 minutes.

4. In a small bowl, blend the brown sugar, mustard, and cannabis tincture. Stir the mixture well to make sure the tincture is evenly distributed.

5. Transfer the bacon to a clean baking sheet and evenly coat each piece with the brown sugar mixture, using the back of a spoon. Return the bacon to the oven for 5 minutes. Turn the bacon over and coat the other side. Cook for 5 more minutes.

6. Set the bacon on a wire rack or paper towels to drain. Store it in an airtight container in the fridge for up to a week.

CANNABIS DOG TREATS

The last time I took my dog Henry to the vet, she said the word *geriatric* as she checked his little hips for pain. Henry just turned eight years old. He doesn't bolt around the dog park like he did when he was a puppy, but he still has his puppy personality, including anxiety about thunderstorms and fireworks. I bought him a ThunderShirt—a snug little sweater to hug him close—but he still trembled and cried and refused to leave my lap during spring storms.

It's fairly common to prescribe glucosamine to keep dogs' joints pain-free and canine antidepressants and antianxiety pills to keep them calm and happy. But dogs can use cannabis to go pharmaceutical-free, too. On our first Fourth of July in Denver, I bought cannabis dog treats at the dispensary, and Henry calmly snoozed through the fireworks. He is a nineteen-pound poodle/cocker spaniel mix, so I give him medicated treats that are tiny but effective. His troubles melt away, he sleeps easily and well, and his life is happier and probably longer because his body isn't processing so much fear.

But we don't want to get our pets high. They don't understand the concept, and the psychoactive effect will increase their anxiety, not reduce it. To keep the THC out of your dog treats, simply skip the decarboxylation step when making doggie edibles. THCA is an analgesic and anti-inflammatory like THC, but without the high, so when we use raw cannabis flower or concentrate, it's THCA, not THC. And remember, too much CBD is a sedative, so if your dog seems too lethargic, cut back a bit on his CBD dose. Small pups need just 5 milligrams of CBD, while bigger dogs can handle 10 milligrams.

Be sure to store your cannabis where your pet can't get to it. If your pet finds your stash and eats too much, you'll know soon enough. He will lose his balance and bladder control and startle easily. Animals will feel the same anxiety that a person does if they consume too much THC. To get them through it, make them comfortable, give them lots of water and treats and tuck a towel or two underneath them, just in case. They'll be fine in a few hours.

This doggie treat recipe can be totally customized to suit your dog's needs. Cook them a little longer for more crunch or pull them from the oven a little early to keep them soft for older teeth. For grain-free treats, use coconut or oat flour, but feel free to use regular white or wheat flour if your dog can tolerate it.

My doggo is a staunch carnivore, so I mix in bacon bits and whatever bacon grease I have in the fridge. I use a cute little bone-shaped cookie cutter to make evenly dosed portions, but you can use anything you like.

Yield: 25 (strong) or 50 (mild) doggie treats

Infusion: Use 3.5 grams of cannabis flower infused in coconut oil (see page 153 for recipe) so that you have about 350 milligrams in the batch. Fifty treats will have 7 milligrams per treat. If you use a 1:1 THC/CBD strain, that means each treat has 3 to 4 milligrams of THC. If your dog weighs less than 10 pounds, break the treats in half. If your dog is more than 100 pounds, give him 2 or 3 treats.

Strain: Use a low-THC, high-CBD or a nondecarboxylated high-THC strain to keep your dog from getting too high.

INGREDIENTS
3.5 grams (for a mild effect) or
   7 grams (for a strong effect)
   cannabis flower
½ cup coconut oil
4 large eggs
1 cup pumpkin puree
½ cup peanut butter
1½ cups flour (coconut or oat for
   gluten-free treats)

EQUIPMENT
Mixing bowl
Hand mixer
Cookie cutter
Baking sheets
Airtight container

1. Infuse the cannabis flower into the coconut oil (see page 153 for recipe).

2. In a mixing bowl, cream together all ingredients with a hand mixer. The dough should be similar in consistency to cookie dough.

3. Roll the dough into 25 to 50 pieces, or roll the dough into one ½-inch-thick slab and cut it into shapes with a cookie cutter. The treats will retain their shape in the oven.

4. Bake the treats on baking sheets at 350°F for 30 minutes or until they are crunchy and brown around the edges.

5. Let them cool at room temperature and store them in an airtight container in a cool, dry place for up to a year.

YOU CAN'T OVERDOSE, BUT YOU MAY OVER*DO*

In 2014, Maureen Dowd went to Denver, bought a medicated chocolate bar, ate too much, got too high, and wrote a newspaper article about the experience. That article set off a chain reaction of new regulations and stricter rules about packaging, labeling, and dosing. Now, marijuana products in every state are clearly labeled with the amount of THC in each package and in each serving. But even with every warning in the world, at some point, someday, it is likely you are going to eat too much THC.

It is very easy to overdo it with edibles. Many edibles have several servings in the package, so if you nibble more than a small bite, you've had three doses. The quality of the marijuana infusion can make an edible more potent, meaning that 20 milligrams of THC in one chocolate bar may make us feel higher than 20 milligrams of THC in another chocolate bar. Some marijuana oils are so potent that a single drop or two is a dose, which means just a few drops can get you too high.

Edibles pose the primary risk for overdoing it. With smoking and vaping, the effects are felt almost immediately, so it is much easier to control your high. But we don't get high from an edible for up to an hour, so there's time to eat too many doses. Plus, everyone's experience is different. Some beginners try 10 milligrams and barely feel high, while others experience 10 milligrams as a hallucinatory panic attack.

Body size and metabolism make a difference; bigger people tend to need bigger doses, but not always. A five-foot-one woman might not feel comfortably high until she's had 50 milligrams of THC, while her six-foot-four husband feels comfortably high with 20 milligrams. To find the right dose, a beginner cannabis user should start low, with 10 milligrams of THC, and increase their dose by 5 to 10 milligrams until they find the dose that relieves their symptoms without side effects—just like any other medication.

A marijuana overdose is not fatal. The activity of the brain stem is not affected by THC, so it is impossible to die from smoking or eating too much weed.

Fans of marijuana say it is perfectly safe and there are no negative side effects to worry about. Opponents of marijuana say it is dangerous and life threatening. Neither is right. There are positive effects when we use cannabis, like pain relief, but there are also a few negative effects from using cannabis. The list is nothing like the lists of negative side effects from prescription medications, but all cannabis users should know what to look out for so they can prevent them. But as long as we stick to a small dose and our hearts aren't on the verge of collapse, we'll be fine. Most side effects fade as you grow from a beginner into an intermediate user and become more tolerant of cannabis.

An hour or two after eating too much weed, you might have a racing heartbeat, paranoia, and anxiety bordering on a panic attack. You might feel bad enough to think you need to go to an urgent care clinic or the emergency room. If you go, they will probably give you a Xanax. The noise, smells, and chaos of the hospital may make your anxiety and paranoia worse. Recovering by staying home, drinking water, eating snacks, and going to bed is a very good option.

The only cure for a marijuana overdose is time. There is nothing we can do to abruptly end a high, so indulge yourself with a lovely session of self-care, including the aforementioned water, delicious snacks, deep breathing, and a long, cozy nap. As long as you keep yourself relaxed, you'll be fine.

To maintain your composure, acknowledge that you feel uncomfortable but it will wear off in a few hours and nothing bad is going to happen. Gently remind yourself that everything will be okay. Take a few deep breaths. If you feel your anxiety increasing, remember what happened, don't blame yourself, and just accept that this will pass soon. The only thing you need to accomplish is getting yourself to bed, just as if you'd come down with an illness. Stop by the kitchen for a snack and a glass of water. Eat anything that tastes good. If you feel dizzy or light-headed, get right into bed. If you aren't tired yet, go to the couch and watch TV until you are ready for sleep. If sha-vasana is your happy place, by all means, roll out your yoga mat and melt into the floor. When I overdo it, I soothe myself with reruns of *The West Wing* until I fall asleep. In the morning, everything is fine. I'm well rested and not hungover.

Negative Side Effects of THC

- Smoking cannabis can cause bronchitis and severe dry mouth. Using a vaporizer eliminates the harm to the lungs, and keeping a fresh glass of cold water, juice, or other non-alcoholic liquid handy keeps your mouth from feeling like a desert.

- Paranoia and anxiety are the biggest negative psychological effects of using or overusing marijuana. If you do start to panic a little, stop smoking or vaping immediately. Stay calm, remember that you aren't doing anything wrong, and take a few deep breaths.

- Like many pleasurable activities, marijuana makes the heart beat a little faster. If your doctor has told you not to step foot on a treadmill or have sex because of your heart, don't use marijuana without medical supervision.

- Marijuana does have physical withdrawal symptoms. Some people experience irritability, trouble sleeping, and a decrease in appetite when they stop using marijuana, but these symptoms are very mild or nonexistent for most people. To experience withdrawal, you need to use a lot of cannabis on a daily basis for a significant amount of time, at least several months, then stop using cannabis. You'll feel a little grumpy, but symptoms don't last beyond a few days.

- Even though you won't die, consuming too much THC feels very uncomfortable and can last for a few hours. It is possible to experience a racing heartbeat, paranoia, anxiety, and disorientation. Supersized doses of THC can also cause shortness of breath, dry mouth, trembling, loss of balance, difficulty moving, nausea, and—potentially—a full-blown panic attack. If this happens, remember to take deep breaths and remind yourself that you'll be just fine soon. Soothe yourself with a hot bath, snacks, lots of water, and the TV.

- The most serious side effect of a marijuana overdose is a spike in blood pressure. You may start to feel light-headed or dizzy, but if you can normally make it through a vigorous workout or the act of lovemaking without having a heart attack, you can enjoy marijuana and even accidentally overdo it and still come out fine on the other side.

Not-Necessarily-Negative Side Effects of THC

When we get high, there are side effects, like short-term memory loss and increased appetite. The cognitive slowdown can be either a positive or a negative effect, depending on why the marijuana is being used in the first place. For someone with PTSD, memory loss is a blessing because they forget about their trauma long enough to relax and fall asleep. The lack of short-term memory while high helps us focus on the task at hand. The rest of the world recedes and the only thing that matters is whatever is happening in the moment. Yoga, cooking, dog walking, swimming, and listening to music are all more enjoyable when we are focused exclusively on them. Because of cognitive impairment and slowed response times while high, tasks where everything that's happening around you must be taken into account—such as operating heavy machinery (including a car) or supervising children—are not well matched with marijuana use.

Once the high wears off, short-term memory returns and everything goes back to normal. Better than normal, in fact. Marijuana works effectively for dementia and Alzheimer's patients, and CBC (one of the lesser-known cannabinoids), in particular, has been shown to grow new brain cells.

The munchies are not an urban legend. THC increases appetite more than any other cannabinoid. The first time you get high, don't be on a diet. Be ready to enjoy food. Not only will marijuana make you hungry, but it also makes food taste amazing. You will eat just for the enjoyment of eating. Have a tasty snack ready to go, like frozen grapes or a bar of your favorite chocolate. Small portions of delicious, rich food keep the French smugly thin, and the same eating habits may keep cannabis users trim, too. Studies have shown that they have a lower BMI than average, and this may be true because of the medicinal compounds in marijuana that lower blood sugar and insulin resistance while improving metabolic function. Marijuana encourages the kind of mindful eating that allows you to appreciate the flavors and textures in food, instead of gobbling down untasted calories. Healthy food tastes better, too. If I have to eat fish and salad for dinner when what I really want is a carton of ice cream, I reach for a joint to make the healthy dinner taste better and feel more satisfying. If getting high gives you the munchies, don't be afraid of it. Use it to eat like the French.

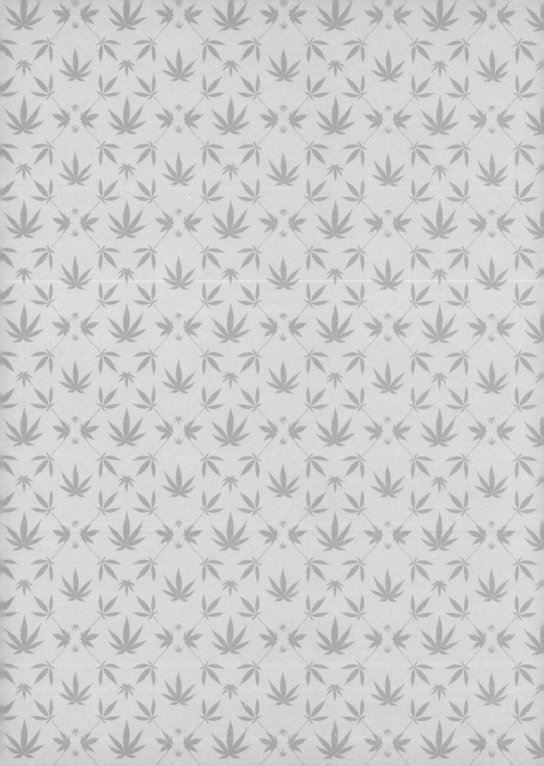

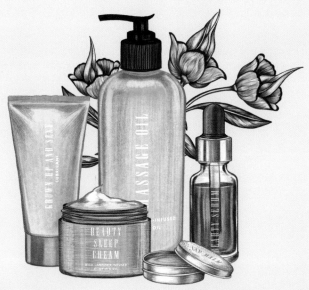

Part Six

TOPICAL CANNABIS– SENSUOUS AND PAIN RELIEVING

Knowing about all the wonderful, medicinal compounds in cannabis and how to inhale and eat it, is going to improve your life significantly. And so will knowing how to take cannabis and rub it right into your skin. Making your own skin treatments and pain creams is easy and a big money saver. The extraction and infusion processes are the same as in baking, and the recipes are easily adaptable, so if you have your own recipes, feel free to use them with the oils and butters.

TOPICALS REDUCE PAIN AND INCREASE BEAUTY

Cannabis improves our appearance by reducing pain, anxiety, and stress, not to mention improving beauty sleep, which makes us look relaxed and happy.

We also get amazing benefits when we apply cannabis directly to the skin. Cannabis-infused creams, lotions, and oils have powerful antiaging benefits in addition to relieving serious skin conditions like eczema, acne, and psoriasis. Healthy skin needs antioxidants; vitamins A, C, and E; and omega-3 and omega-6 fatty acids. Cannabis is loaded with all of them. Marijuana is anti-inflammatory and antifungal, and clinical research has shown that antioxidants in marijuana support lipid production, which regulates the oil in skin and controls acne and dry patches. The skin, hair follicles, sweat glands, and sebaceous glands have receptors for cannabinoids and terpenes to lock into and work their magic. Creams and lotions won't get us high (because the THC absorbed by the skin does not enter the bloodstream), but they will give us the best skin we've ever had.

Dispensaries now have small selections of cannabis-infused creams, but these creams are formulated for pain, not great skin. Someday soon, cannabis producers and beauty experts will get together and create fabulous moisturizers and eye creams for various skin types in pretty packaging that we just pick up at the dispensary, but until that day, we have to make our own.

The good news is that it is very easy to whip up luxurious beauty treatments at home, with just a couple of ingredients.

Guidelines for Great Topicals

- Pain relief topicals require more cannabis than beauty treatments do.

- Cannabis for skin doesn't need to be decarboxylated. The anti-inflammatory properties of THCA and CBDA are just as beneficial in skin creams and oils as THC and CBD. In the dispensary, look for creams and lotions that have a full range of cannabinoids, including THC, CBD, THCA, and CBDA.

- The recipes in this book are for cannabis flower, but it is very easy to substitute cannabis concentrate in topicals. Here's the trick. Melt the concentrate in the oven at 250 degrees Fahrenheit for 20 minutes. During the last few minutes, melt the rest of your ingredients in the microwave. Then, stir the melted concentrate into the melted ingredients and continue the steps of the recipe. This is the only way I make topicals now. When the dispensary has a sale on wax, shatter, or live resin, I stock up. When I need to make a pain cream or replace an empty bottle of moisturizing oil, I grab one of the cheap grams of concentrate and melt it.

- DIY topicals do not require any special equipment beyond a collection of mason jars and pretty bottles and containers to store oils, serums, salves, and creams. Oils work well in 1- and 2-ounce bottles with dropper tops or sprayers for a fine-mist application. I pick up pretty, colorful glass bottles and jars at flea markets, garage sales, Goodwill, and big box stores. Look online for spray bottles and lip balm tubes.

- I love scented lotions, but my skin does not. If you have a collection of essential oils and scents, get them out and play with your topical oils, creams, and lotions. If you don't, or you prefer fragrance-free skin products, skip the scents. The scent of cannabis usually does not come through in topicals—the butters and oils do a good job of covering it up.

- Sephora and Whole Foods have lots of hemp oil products. This is great because hemp seed oil is wonderfully moisturizing. But cannabinoids and terpenes are only in cannabis, not hemp. Skin treatments with cannabis can relieve pain, soothe aches and sore muscles, reduce inflammation, and heal severe skin conditions. Topicals made from marijuana can only be sold in dispensaries, not online, so they're harder to get—but worth it.

- Emu oil helps cannabinoids sink into the skin and get to work. Emu oil is the darling of the marijuana topical world. The claim is that emu oil penetrates the layers of the skin more than other oils, which, in theory, would carry more cannabinoids through the skin and directly to the receptors of the endocannabinoid system. I don't know if this is true, but when I make creams and oils with emu oil, my skin looks amazing, so I keep using it.

- Make sure to use fresh oils and add drops of vitamin E to every topical recipe. Vitamin E adds shelf life to topicals so they don't go rancid.

- Beware of coconut oil, particularly on your face. I tried it, thinking it would make my skin look better. Within a week my nose was one giant clogged pore, and my cheeks were covered in flaming red, painful acne. Eventually, I tried a new concoction: high-CBD CO_2 oil stirred into warmed argan oil. I rubbed a dropperful of infused oil into my palms and coated my face, neck, and hands with it. Immediately, I felt like Cleopatra. My skin felt perfectly balanced for the first time in my life. The next day, my face felt fixed. Clear pores, no redness, and all the acne dried up and disappeared in a week. Argan oil is my magic oil, so I use it in everything. I combine it with beeswax for lip balm and whip it with shea butter for creams. If you find your own magic oil, stick with it.

- Topicals are made from natural butters and oils, and some are better for our skin than others. *Comedogenic* means pore clogging, while *noncomedogenic* means pore clearing. There

COMEDOGENIC RATING SYSTEM

0 = LOW PORE CLOGGING

Argan Oil: 0
Avocado Oil: 3
Cocoa Butter: 4
Coconut Butter: 4
Coconut Oil: 4
Emu Oil: 1
Grape Seed Oil: 1
Hemp Seed Oil: 0
Jojoba Oil: 2
Linseed (Flaxseed) Oil: 4

5 = HIGH PORE CLOGGING

Mango Butter: 2
Mink Oil: 3
Neem Oil: 1
Olive Oil: 2
Rosehip Oil: 1
Sesame Oil: 3
Shea Butter: 1
Sunflower Oil: 0
Sweet Almond Oil: 2
Wheat Germ Oil: 5

is a comedogenic rating system for oils on a scale of zero to five. Zero means the oil won't clog pores, even for oily skin. A rating of five means the oil will clog pores for every skin type. Oils with ratings of two, three, and four will clog pores for some skin types. I have sensitive, oily skin that breaks out at anything, so I stick to level zero or one oils. Most skin types are just fine with level two oils, and very dry skin can handle level four without breaking out. When I make topicals for friends, I use the comedogenic rating scale to choose the right butters and oils for their skin types and body parts. I use level three or four oils in foot creams and foot oils. My elbows turn into Brillo pads in winter, so I make a custom-blended coconut oil to soften them up. Go low on the scale for summer face moisturizers, acne, and oily skin.

Oils and Serums

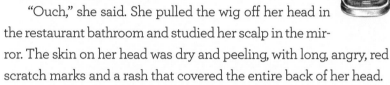

I was having lunch with my friend Sarah when she stuck her fingers in her platinum-blond wig and winced as she scratched her scalp. Chemo was over, the prognosis was good, she didn't have another doctor's appointment scheduled for six months, and her hair was growing back.

"Ouch," she said. She pulled the wig off her head in the restaurant bathroom and studied her scalp in the mirror. The skin on her head was dry and peeling, with long, angry, red scratch marks and a rash that covered the entire back of her head.

After lunch I went home and mixed up a bottle of oil. I brought it to Sarah's house and rubbed the infused oil into her damaged scalp. She almost purred as her shoulders dropped and her eyes closed. Sarah rubbed the oil into her head every night, and within a week the rash and the wig were gone. Her scalp was now a smooth cue ball of clear skin.

"You look good, lady. All glowy. Are you pregnant?" I asked at our next lunch.

"Oh god, I hope not," she said. "I'm over forty and over babies. It's the oil. I'm using it on my face, too." She waved a hand under her eyes. "I don't know where they went, but the bags under my eyes are gone."

I've found that jojoba oil doesn't leave a shine, so we can use this serum during the day and under makeup. For antiaging, rosehip oil is rich and nourishing with vitamins A, C, and E, while avocado oil boosts collagen production. When the oils are warmed, they blend smoothly with the marijuana concentrate or tincture.

RADIANT GLOW SERUM

Yield: 2 ounces of oil

Infusion: This serum is made by infusing 3.5 grams of cannabis flower into jojoba oil (see page 153 for recipe).

Strain: Choose a high-potency 1:1 THC/CBD strain and decarb for 30 minutes rather than an hour (see page 143 for recipe) for a full range of cannabinoids.

To use: Put a few drops on fingertips and gently massage into skin.

INGREDIENTS

3.5 grams (for a mild effect) or 7 grams (for a strong effect) cannabis flower

2 tablespoons (1 ounce) jojoba oil

2 tablespoons (1 ounce) emu oil

10 drops vitamin E oil

5 drops lemon essential oil

5 drops neroli essential oil

EQUIPMENT

Small heatproof bowl

Whisk

Airtight bottle

1. Infuse the cannabis flower into the jojoba oil (see page 153 for recipe).

2. In a small heatproof bowl, warm the jojoba and emu oils in 30-second increments in the microwave.

3. Add the remaining ingredients to the warmed oils.

4. Whisk and cool the mixture to room temperature.

5. Store the serum in an airtight bottle in a cool, dry place for up to 6 months.

HOLY ANOINTING OIL

In biblical times, cannabis had less THC and more CBD than it has today. Basically, it was the perfect medicine for epileptics and an amazing pain reducer. In Mark 6:13, Jesus and his disciples "cast out many devils, and anointed with oil many that were sick, and healed them." Someone having a seizure in biblical times would terrify most people into believing in demons, and if Jesus came along and gave them a dose of oil, stopped the seizures, and chased away demons, I'd be a believer, too.

A recipe in Exodus calls for cannabis, olive oil, myrrh, and cinnamon. I've created it as an olive oil tincture. I don't love cinnamon, so I usually substitute other herbs and flavors like ginger, lemon balm, garlic, rosemary, peppermint, cayenne, chamomile, and angelica. Use either olive oil or fractionated coconut oil, depending on personal preference and taste.

Holy anointing oil can be eaten as a tincture or rubbed into skin for pain relief.

Yield: ¼ cup of oil

Infusion: This oil is made by infusing 3.5 grams of cannabis flower into olive oil (see page 153 for recipe).

Strain: Choose a high-potency 1:1 THC/CBD strain and decarb for 30 minutes rather than an hour (see page 143 for recipe) for a full range of cannabinoids.

To use: Put a few drops on fingertips and rub into skin. Or swallow the oil as an edible.

INGREDIENTS
3.5 grams (for a mild effect) or
   7 grams (for a strong effect)
   cannabis flower
¼ cup olive oil
10 drops vitamin E oil
10 drops cinnamon oil
10 drops frankincense oil

EQUIPMENT
Small heatproof bowl
Whisk
Airtight bottle or jar

1. Infuse cannabis flower into olive oil (see page 153 for recipe).

2. Pour the infused olive oil into a heatproof bowl and place it in the microwave. Heat it on high in 30-second bursts, stirring between each burst. Stop when it's noticeably warm but not hot.

3. Add the remaining ingredients to the bowl of warm olive oil.

4. Stir well. Cool at room temperature.

5. Store the finished oil in an airtight bottle or jar in a cool, dry place for up to 6 months.

CANNABIS SUPPOSITORIES

Suppositories are the cannabis product that patients and budtenders want to talk about the most, and for good reason. Suppositories are the most effective way to take any medication because there are numerous pathways to the bloodstream in the rectum, so cannabinoids like THC and CBD are absorbed almost immediately.

For most of us, if we eat 100 milligrams of THC, we get really, really, uncomfortably high. But 100 milligrams in a suppository is a much milder high. For patients who need hundreds of milligrams a day of THC, suppositories are the best way to get them without literally smoking weed all day.

Suppositories are also the easiest infused products to make at home. We simply need cocoa butter and molds, which are easy to find online. Most suppository molds are around 2 milliliters each. Since there are 15 milliliters in an ounce (2 tablespoons) of cocoa butter, we can make 15 suppositories with ¼ cup of cocoa butter. If 7 grams of flower or 1 gram of concentrate is infused, each of the 15 suppositories will have 50 milligrams. If you want 100 milligrams in each suppository, double the grams of flower while using the same amount of cocoa butter.

Yield: Fifteen 2-milliliter suppositories

Infusion: For a mild suppository, infuse 7 grams of marijuana flower or 1 gram concentrate into the cocoa butter. For a stronger suppository, infuse 14 grams of flower or 2 grams of concentrate into the cocoa butter.

The butter recipe on page 148 applies to cocoa butter as well. Follow it, simply substituting the same amount of cocoa butter for dairy butter.

Strain: Choose a strain with more than 20 percent total potency.

To use: Carefully peel the mold from the suppository. Lie down and gently insert into the rectum. Stay prone and relaxed for 30 minutes while the butter melts and is absorbed by the body.

INGREDIENTS

3.5 grams (for a mild effect) or 7 grams (for a strong effect) cannabis flower

¼ cup (two ounces) cocoa butter

EQUIPMENT

Small heatproof bowl

Squeeze bottle

15 suppository molds

Airtight container

1. Infuse the cannabis flower into the cocoa butter (see page 148 for general butter recipe).

2. In a small heatproof bowl, microwave cocoa butter in 30-second increments until completely melted.

3. Pour the mixture into a squeeze bottle. Shake well. Carefully fill each mold with the infused butter.

4. Cool the suppositories at room temperature overnight. Store them in an airtight container in a cool, dry place for up to a year.

Solid Lotion Bars

I was standing at the counter in a dispensary in Springfield, Illinois, when the budtender started talking to the customer in line behind me.

"This is Nikki. She made that topical bar you love so much," she said.

"Oh! Thank you so much! You saved my life!" The man behind me, who was wearing a Harley-Davidson T-shirt and had long hair, had tears in his eyes as he shook my hand. "I feel so much better when I use it. It's the only reason I'm standing up right now!"

I knew what he meant because I didn't fully appreciate the healing benefits of marijuana-infused lotion until I fractured my spine. Rubbing a topical bar on my back made the difference between standing up and lying on the floor with muscle spasms.

It is a struggle for arthritic hands to open tiny jars of salve or squeeze bottles of lotion. Sometimes just removing a cap can be painful. A solid lotion bar, on the other hand, requires no packaging and can sit on the bathroom counter. Simply pick it up and rub it where it hurts. Bars are solid like soap, but when they are rubbed on the skin, they leave a light layer of medicated, moisturizing lotion.

Lotion bars don't require a mixer, and with a little creativity can be made into any shape you like. Use soap molds, small ramekins, or a muffin pan for a mold. I use small plastic food containers to make palm-sized bars.

For a softer bar that easily and quickly melts onto the skin, use a little less beeswax and a little more liquid oil. If your bars melt too quickly, especially in summer, use a little more beeswax and a bit less oil. You can also store them in the fridge for more solidity.

HAPPY BODY BAR

A solid lotion bar is a great option for muscle pain because it's so easy to rub the bar wherever it hurts. Keep one in your gym bag for sore muscles and one in your bathroom for daily aches and pains. Use more cannabis for more pain relief. For my sciatic nerve pain, I add 2 grams of CO_2 oil because nerve pain is tough and a milder topical won't work. I use this double-dose bar on my right leg, hip, and back when I've been chairbound all day. I've had severe arthritis patients need the double-dose bar, too.

Emu oil helps the cannabinoids sink down into the skin. Peppermint and eucalyptus add an extra tingle and smell much better than other medicinal pain creams.

Yield: Two 3-ounce bars

Infusion: These bars are made by infusing cannabis flower into emu oil (see page 153 for recipe).

Strain: Choose a high-potency 1:1 THC/CBD strain and decarb for 30 minutes rather than an hour (see page 143 for recipe) for a full range of cannabinoids.

To use: Hold the bar against the skin to warm it up, then rub the bar over the area to coat the skin in a light layer of lotion.

INGREDIENTS

3.5 grams (for a mild effect) or 7 grams (for a strong effect) cannabis flower

¼ cup emu oil

¼ cup beeswax

¼ cup cocoa butter

5 drops vitamin E oil

5 drops peppermint essential oil

5 drops eucalyptus essential oil

EQUIPMENT

Large heatproof bowl

Whisk

Molds

Parchment paper or plastic wrap

1. Infuse the cannabis flower into the emu oil (see page 153 for recipe).

2. Put the beeswax and cocoa butter in a large heatproof bowl and place in the microwave. Heat in 30-second increments, whisking in between, until fully melted. Add infused emu oil, vitamin E, and peppermint and eucalyptus oils, and whisk until well blended.

3. Pour the mixture into molds and let the bars cool at room temperature until they are solid. Wrap the bars in parchment paper or plastic wrap for storage. Store them in a cool, dry place for up to a year.

Whipped Creams

Sometimes the smooth texture of a lotion or cream is better than an oil, and they are very easy to make. Rich, luxurious creams just need butter or beeswax for a touch of solidity and a hand mixer to do the whipping. It's also important to remember that the cream won't cream up properly unless the entire batch is cold, so make sure you don't try to whip too early.

Creams are infused with medicated oil, concentrate, or tincture. The number of milligrams is not as important as it is with edibles, so with topicals we use the theory of more is better. Concentrates like wax, shatter, and CO_2 oil have more milligrams than infused oils or tincture, but they need to be melted into butters to ensure even distribution throughout the cream.

BEAUTY SLEEP CREAM

This rich cream softens and smooths skin while you sleep. I always make it with lavender, which helps induce sleep. Apply a thin layer to your face, neck, chest, and hands before bed. Shea butter and olive oil combine for an overnight deep-conditioning treatment.

Yield: 4 ounces of cream

Infusion: This cream is made by infusing cannabis flower into olive oil (see page 153 for recipe).

Strain: Choose a high-potency 1:1 THC/CBD strain and decarb for 30 minutes rather than an hour (see page 143 for recipe) for a full range of cannabinoids.

To use: Before bed, massage lightly into face like regular cream.

INGREDIENTS

3.5 grams (for a mild effect) or
   7 grams (for a strong effect)
   cannabis flower
¼ cup olive oil
¼ cup shea butter
1 teaspoon vitamin E oil
5 drops lavender essential oil
2 tablespoons liquid lecithin

EQUIPMENT

Small heatproof bowl
Whisk
Immersion blender or beater
Spatula
Airtight jar

1. Infuse the cannabis flower into the olive oil (see page 153 for recipe).

2. Place the shea butter in a small heatproof bowl and heat in the microwave at full power in 30-second bursts. Add the rest of the ingredients and whisk for several minutes before cooling in the fridge for an hour.

3. Using an immersion blender or beater, whip the mixture into a creamy texture. Allow the mixture to come to room temperature.

4. With a spatula, scrape down the sides of the bowl and whip again so that all the cream is whipped.

5. Store the cream in an airtight jar in a cool, dry place for up to a year.

FOOT-REVIVING CREAM

I am miserable when my feet hurt, and high heels make me homicidal. On a lifelong quest for happy feet, I've tried every clunky, ugly, "comfortable" shoe I can find, and still, my feet ache. Women abuse their feet every day in high heels and bad shoes, and we pay for it with muscle cramps, plantar fasciitis, bunions, cracked heels, and swollen ankles. Rubbing marijuana-infused cream into those barking dogs relieves pain and makes skin smooth and soft.

This is an intentionally gloppy, greasy cream. Petroleum jelly (Vaseline) heals cracked heels and calluses, while peppermint and tea tree refresh and invigorate the skin.

Yield: 4 ounces of cream

Infusion: This cream is made by infusing cannabis flower into coconut oil (see page 153 for recipe).

Strain: Choose a high-potency 1:1 THC/CBD strain and decarb for 30 minutes rather than an hour (see page 143 for recipe) for a full range of cannabinoids.

To use: At the end of a long day, take a bath, shower, or foot soak and give your feet a quick scrub, then massage a quarter-sized dollop of cream into your feet before pulling on a pair of thick socks. Lie on the floor with your legs up against the wall, or at least put your feet up on the couch, higher than your heart for a circulation boost. Rest. In the morning, pull off the socks. Feet will be soft, revived, and ready for another day.

INGREDIENTS
3.5 grams (for a mild effect) or
   7 grams (for a strong effect)
   cannabis flower
¼ cup coconut oil
¼ cup cocoa butter
5 drops vitamin E oil
5 drops peppermint oil extract
5 drops tea tree essential oil

2 tablespoons lecithin
¼ cup petroleum jelly

EQUIPMENT
Small heatproof bowl
Whisk
Hand mixer
Spatula
4-ounce airtight container

1. Infuse the cannabis flower into the coconut oil (see page 153 for recipe).

2. Melt the cocoa butter in a small heatproof bowl in the microwave in 30-second increments. Add the remaining ingredients, except for the petroleum jelly, and whisk until thoroughly blended. Cool in the fridge for an hour.

3. Add the petroleum jelly and use the hand mixer to whip the mixture to a creamy texture. With a spatula, scrape down the sides of the bowl to whip all the cream.

4. Scoop the cream into an airtight container and store it in a cool, dry place for up to a year.

TIPS FOR WHIPPING CREAM

- To whip oils and butters into cream, use a blender, immersion blender, or mixer. If I'm making a tiny batch, I use the mixer. If I'm making a double batch, I pull out the immersion blender. For a big, home-made-Christmas-gifts-for-everyone-sized batch, I use the blender.

- The most important thing to remember is not to whip the mixture until it is cooled. Warm oils and butters won't whip up into a smooth cream. Leave the mixture in the fridge until completely and totally cooled.

- Liquid lecithin is an emulsifier and makes creams, lotions, and body butters feel richer and more luxurious.

VANILLA-MINT LIP BALM

Wrinkled, dry lips make me look like a disapproving pearl clutcher. Antiaging lip balm maintains smooth, plump, and moisturized lips. You can find DIY lip balm tube molds or tins at craft stores, beauty supply stores, and online. Use a squeeze bottle to get the melted balm into the molds without a mess. If you make these in winter, use a touch more oil and a bit less beeswax so they don't dry out and crack in cold weather. In the summer, use a touch more beeswax and a bit less oil so they don't melt in the heat.

Yield: 10 to 14 tubes or tins, depending on size

Infusion: These balms are made by infusing cannabis flower into sweet almond oil (see page 153 for recipe).

Strain: Choose a high-potency 1:1 THC/CBD strain and decarb for 30 minutes rather than an hour (see page 143 for recipe) for a full range of cannabinoids.

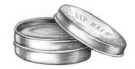

To use: Apply directly to lips.

INGREDIENTS

3.5 grams (for a mild effect) or 7 grams (for a strong effect) cannabis flower

2 tablespoons (1 ounce) sweet almond oil

5 tablespoons (2.5 ounces) beeswax

5 drops vitamin E oil

10 drops peppermint flavoring

10 drops vanilla flavoring

EQUIPMENT

Small heatproof bowl

Whisk

Squeeze bottle

Lip balm tubes or tins

1. Infuse the cannabis flower into the sweet almond oil (see page 153 for recipe).

2. Microwave the beeswax in a heatproof bowl at full power in 30-second bursts until melted.

3. Add the infused sweet almond oil and the remaining ingredients. Stir well until the mixture is completely blended.

4. Pour into a squeeze bottle. Carefully fill the tubes or tins. Let the lip balm mixtures cool uncovered at room temperature and store them in a cool, dry place for up to a year.

Grooming for Men

Men like to look good, too, so we have a few options for them. The best thing about cannabis-infused grooming products is that men will actually use them.

MUSTACHE WAX

This is a light-hold, conditioning wax to moisturize the skin and keep mustache hairs smoothed neatly in place. Most men I know prefer it unscented, because the product sits right under the nose, but if your man is into scent, go ahead and add a few drops. This is also a basic lip balm and eyebrow gel, so make one for yourself, too. There are lots of cute lip balm tins available to store these in.

Yield: 2 to 4 small tins of wax

Infusion: This wax is made by infusing cannabis flower into argan oil (see page 153 for recipe).

Strain: Choose a high-potency 1:1 THC/CBD strain and decarb for 30 minutes rather than an hour (see page 143 for recipe) for a full range of cannabinoids.

To use: Lightly apply to mustache, beard, and eyebrows to keep in place.

INGREDIENTS
3.5 grams (for a mild effect) or
   7 grams (for a strong effect)
   cannabis flower
2 tablespoons (1 ounce) argan oil
3 tablespoons (1 to 1½ ounces)
   beeswax
5 drops vitamin E oil
2–4 drops of scent, if desired

EQUIPMENT
Small heatproof bowl
Whisk
Squeeze bottle or spoon
Lip balm tins

1. Infuse the cannabis flower into the argan oil (see page 153 for recipe).

2. Microwave the beeswax in 30-second increments in a heatproof bowl until melted. Add the cannabis-infused argan oil and the vitamin E oil to the melted beeswax. Stir well until all ingredients are completely blended.

3. Carefully fill the tins. You can spoon it into the tins or use a squeeze bottle.

4. Let the wax cool at room temperature and store the tins in a cool, dry place for up to a year.

WINTER BEARD OIL

Beards need more grooming than clean-shaven faces, and in the depths of winter, the skin underneath those shaggy beards needs attention, too. This oil can also be used to keep scalp skin moisturized and protected from winter winds. I make this beard oil with sweet almond oil for deep moisturizing, but feel free to use a lighter oil for oily skin or a heavier oil for extremely dry skin.

Yield: 30 applications

Infusion: This oil is made by infusing cannabis flower into sweet almond oil (see page 153 for recipe).

Strain: Choose a high-potency 1:1 THC/CBD strain and decarb for 30 minutes rather than an hour (see page 143 for recipe) for a full range of cannabinoids.

To use: Squeeze a dropperful into palm. Rub hands together, then rub into beard.

INGREDIENTS
3.5 grams (for a mild effect) or
   7 grams (for a strong effect)
   cannabis flower
3 tablespoons (1.5 ounces) sweet
   almond oil
5 drops sandalwood essential oil
10 drops vitamin E oil

EQUIPMENT
Small heatproof bowl
Whisk
1-ounce bottle with dropper top

1. Infuse the cannabis flower into the sweet almond oil (see page 153 for recipe).

2. Combine and microwave the sweet almond and sandalwood oils in a heatproof bowl in 30-second bursts at full power until warm. Add the vitamin E. Stir the mixture well until it is completely blended.

3. Let the mixture cool at room temperature and pour it into a 1-ounce bottle with a dropper top. Store the beard oil in a cool, dry place for up to a year.

Massage Oils and Personal Lubricants

Women who use cannabis already know this, but it might surprise a lot of men when they find out that cannabis is basically Viagra for women. When women get high, they feel relaxed and happy. Stress disappears, and they forget about their troubles and focus on the good feelings of the moment. Getting high is the easiest way to get in the mood to fool around.

If I created a product called Relationship Therapy in a Box and sold it in dispensaries, I would include two chocolate edibles with 20 milligrams THC/CBD, a small bottle of cannabis-infused lubricant, and two pre-rolled joints (indica, 15 percent THC). And the instructions for orgasmic meditation.

Orgasmic meditation is when a partner spends fifteen minutes stroking the clitoris of their partner. That's it. The goal is not orgasm, but connection to another person and feeling good. For women, the meditation builds intimacy, trust, and an emotional connection. For their partner, the meditation allows them to focus on empathy and an emotional connection. For cannabis users, it gives the THC a chance to kick in.

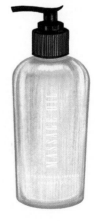

Start with the edibles. Eat them first, so they can have thirty to forty-five minutes to kick in. Go for a low-dose edible with an equal amount of THC and CBD to get rid of anxiety and relax. Smoke or vape an inhalation or two for an immediate mood boost. Choose a medium-potency THC to avoid anxiety, and an indica for a lovely body high.

Then get into bed with your cannabis-infused lube or massage oil and settle into the orgasmic meditation. Massage oils and lubricants take anywhere from twenty to thirty minutes before they become effective and tingly, so take your time.

Oil-based lube feels good but makes condoms less effective. Always use a water-based lube with condoms.

CHERRY MASSAGE OIL

Infused coconut oil can be eaten, rubbed into the skin as a topical, or rubbed into intimate places. But it doesn't taste great, so we add flavor oils. Sweet and fruity flavors are always popular, but feel free to get exotic. In a pinch, grab the vanilla extract. Try peppermint oil extract for a little extra kick. Some dispensaries sell flavored coconut oil, so ask your budtender if it's available.

Yield: ¼ cup of oil

Infusion: This oil is made by infusing cannabis flower into coconut oil (see page 153 for recipe).

Strain: A strong THC level works best for this oil, so decarboxylate fully for an hour.

To use: Store in a small, squeezable plastic bottle. Shake well before use. Apply a few drops to your fingertips, then gently massage wherever your partner tells you to.

INGREDIENTS
3.5 grams (for a mild effect) or
   7 grams (for a strong effect)
   cannabis flower
¼ cup (2 ounces) fractionated
   coconut oil

20 drops cherry flavoring
10 drops vitamin E oil

EQUIPMENT
Small bowl
Whisk
Small, squeezable plastic bottle

1. Infuse the cannabis flower into the coconut oil (see page 153 for recipe).

2. Place the infused coconut oil in a small bowl and add the flavoring and vitamin E. Stir well.

3. Store the mixture in a small, squeezable plastic bottle in a cool, dark place for up to 6 months.

GROWN AND SEXY LUBRICANT

Smart grown-ups take good care of themselves, which means using a water-based lubricant that is safe to use with condoms. Add a touch more cornstarch or arrowroot powder and cook for an extra minute or two for a thicker gel. If you prefer a thinner, more liquid consistency, use a pinch less cornstarch or arrowroot powder and remove from heat as soon as it boils. If you can't find absinthe, substitute moonshine, vodka or Everclear. The chocolate extract is for flavoring. It pairs well with absinthe, but feel free to choose your favorite flavors.

Yield: ½ cup of lubricant

Infusion: This lubricant is made by infusing cannabis flower into absinthe (see page 157 for recipe).

Strain: Go for full-strength THC and decarb for the full hour.

To use: Store in a small, squeezable plastic bottle. Apply a few drops to fingertips, then gently massage wherever your partner tells you to.

INGREDIENTS
3.5 grams (for a mild effect) or 7 grams (for a strong effect) cannabis flower
1 ounce absinthe
½ cup water
2 teaspoons cornstarch or arrowroot powder
1 teaspoon chocolate extract
10 drops vitamin E oil

EQUIPMENT
Small saucepan
Whisk
Small, squeezable plastic bottle

1. Infuse cannabis flower into absinthe (see page 157 for recipe).

2. In a small saucepan, bring the water and the cornstarch or arrowroot powder to a boil. Remove the mixture from the heat and add the absinthe, chocolate extract, and vitamin E. Whisk the mixture well and let it cool to room temperature.

3. Store the lubricant in a small, squeezable plastic bottle or jar in a cool, dark place for up to 6 months.

THINGS TO REMEMBER

- When making your own skin cream, aim for around 25 to 50 milligrams of THC/CBD per ounce of cream. With oils, infuse 100 to 350 milligrams per ounce of oil.

- THC, CBD, THCA, and CBDA are all anti-inflammatory. Look for topicals with a full range of cannabinoids.

- Use or make more potent topicals for pain relief, and milder topicals for beauty treatments and daily moisturizers.

- Keep coconut oil away from your face. Use it on rough, dry patches, like heels and elbows.

GLOSSARY/DISPENSARY SLANG—
A PARTIAL LIST

Blunt—While joints are rolled with cigarette paper, blunts are rolled with cigar paper. They are larger and usually are shared at parties.

Bogart—To hold on to a joint for too long before passing it to the next person. Derived from the iconic image of Humphrey Bogart with a cigarette firmly held in his mouth.

Bubble hash—This hash can be vaped or smoked. To produce bubble hash, cannabis is agitated in ice water and then dried into a powdery concentrate.

Bubbler—Bubblers are miniature bongs that are approximately the size of a small glass pipe. Portable and powerful.

Bud—The flowering buds of the cannabis plant are the mainstay of recreational consumption. Leaves and trim—the leftover parts of the plant—have cannabinoids and terpenes that can be used in medicine, but they are not nearly as potent as the buds.

Cashed—Means "empty"; used when all the cannabis has been consumed from a bong, pipe, or vaporizer. "This bowl is cashed. Want to pack another?"

Chronic—A slang term for cannabis with hip-hop origins. Coined by Snoop Dogg, musician and producer, he claims to have misunderstood the word *hydroponic*, thinking it was *hydrochronic*, and shortened it to *chronic*.

Cola—The site on the cannabis plant where the bud blooms; topmost bud is the main cola.

Cotton mouth—Dry mouth that occurs during or after cannabis consumption. Some strains are more drying than others.

Diesel—Cannabis strains with an aroma of gasoline and the feel of a sativa—energizing and cerebral—have Diesel genetics. Sour Diesel is the most well-known Diesel strain.

Dugout—A small box specially designed for holding a one-hitter and a small amount of cannabis; can be kept in a purse and used on the go.

Ganja—Sanskrit for hemp and the preferred name for cannabis among Rastafarians. Also called *ganj*.

Grinder—Like a specialized pepper mill, a grinder is a twistable cylindrical device filled with prongs or tines that break up clumps of cannabis for easy, smooth consumption.

Haze—A very old sativa strain that shows up in today's Blue Dream, Super Lemon Haze, Super Silver Haze, Amnesia Haze, Neville's Haze, and Ghost Train Haze strains. A very potent sativa.

Hot box—Filling a small, closed space with marijuana smoke to amplify the smoke's effects is called *hot boxing*.

Kush—From the Hindu Kush mountains of Afghanistan and Pakistan, Kush strains are powerful indicas that encourage relaxation and sleep.

Muggle-head—In the Harry Potter series, muggles are people without magic. In the 1920s, cannabis smokers were called muggle-heads. *Muggles* is synonymous with *reefer*, meaning either cannabis or a joint.

Nug—Short for *nugget*; a single cannabis bud.

Nug run/trim run—When a concentrate is made from pure cannabis buds, it's called *nug run*. Concentrates made from the entire plant—buds, but also sugar leaves and trim—are called *trim run*.

OG—In hip-hop, *OG* means Original Gangster, but with regard to cannabis, it also means Ocean Grown (as opposed to "mountain-grown" cannabis, a variety of powerful strains from Central Asia). OG Kush is a popular strain from the '90s that has been used to breed many other strains.

One-hitter—A small, economical pipe that holds just enough cannabis for one or two inhalations.

Pack a bowl—Slang expression for filling a smoking device with ground cannabis.

Pinner—A very thin joint.

Popcorn buds—Smaller, less potent buds than colas that grow lower on the stem of a cannabis plant.

Puff, puff, pass—The unspoken-but-typical practice when smoking or vaping with others. You take two inhalations and pass the joint, pipe, or blunt to the next person. If you've had enough and the group is still smoking, you can simply pass.

Rig—Also called a *dab rig*, this is a bong-like device for vaping cannabis concentrates.

Roach—The nub of a consumed joint and the most difficult to smoke. Dispensary joints have filter tips that make roaches extinct.

Shake—Cannabis flower buds are ground into shake, so they can be packed into rolling papers and pipes.

Sploof—Sploofs are filters that dampen the smell of marijuana. Stuff a dryer sheet into a cardboard tube or a plastic bottle with one end removed and exhale smoke through the tube. You can cover the end with a sock for added filtration.

Trim run—See *Nug run*.

Wake and bake—To get high in the morning. "I have the day off tomorrow. Want to wake and bake before brunch?"

SUGGESTED READING LIST

These days I grow and sell marijuana, but I am a bookseller at heart. Everything I know, I learned from books. I wrote this book because there was nothing that explained everything my mom needed to know about medical marijuana in a way that she would understand, so I wrote one for her. These are the books I used to do it. They taught me how to cook, how to think about food, and what tastes good together. They taught me how to grow, cook, and smoke weed like a lady.

The Art of Simple Food, and everything else Alice Waters has ever written

The Botany of Desire: A Plant's-Eye View of the World by Michael Pollan

Butter: A Rich History by Elaine Khosrova

Cannabis Pharmacy: The Practical Guide to Medical Marijuana by Michael Backes

The Flavor Bible by Karen Page and Andrew Dornenburg

The Great Book of Chocolate by David Lebovitz

How to Cook Everything by Mark Bittman

Make the Bread, Buy the Butter by Jennifer Reese

Marijuana Growers Handbook: Your Complete Guide for Medical and Personal Marijuana Cultivation by Ed Rosenthal

Marijuana Horticulture: The Indoor/Outdoor Medical Grower's Bible by Jorge Cervantes

My Master Recipes by Patricia Wells

The Perfect Scoop by David Lebovitz

The Pot Book: A Complete Guide to Cannabis by
    Julie Holland, MD
Real Fast Desserts by Nigel Slater
Salt, Fat, Acid, Heat by Samin Nosrat
Stoned: A Doctor's Case for Medical Marijuana by
    David Casarett, MD
Weed the People: The Future of Legal Marijuana in America
    by Bruce Barcott

ACKNOWLEDGMENTS

Writing this book was a group effort, so there are many people I'd like to thank for their time, talent, and effort.

Dan Lazar is the most handsome and charming literary agent in New York, and a wonderful old friend.

Mary Ellen O'Neill knew it was time for women and weed, and she shaped this book into the gem that it is. Everything good about it is because of her.

Thank you to everyone else at Workman, including Suzie Bolotin, Becky Terhune, Jessica Rozler, Barbara Peragine, Lathea Williams, and Cindy Lee, and the wonderful sales force. Lisel Ashlock deserves special thanks for making the book so beautiful with her lovely illustrations.

Tom Colclasure is the best mentor and business partner anyone could ever wish for. He is a gentle soul with the heart of a lion. Special thanks to Kathy Readnour for her compassion and kindness. I am eternally grateful to Mike, the best marijuana grower I have ever known. And Danielle, who proves that edibles chefs should run the world. I will always be grateful to Allison Braden for sharing her pharmacist magic and teaching me how to make suppositories.

Thank you to the Illinois Department of Agriculture inspectors for their patience and good humor.

Thank you to the mountain growers who don't want their names in print.

Thank you to my taste testers, recipe checkers, and guinea pigs—Erin Kasten, Monica Taylor, Rich Barbieri, Amanda Harvey Foley, Beckie Miller Jacobs, Salvatore LoForte, Amanda

Galloway, Steven Smith, Kate Stewart, Spencer Gould, and my mom and her friends.

I am grateful to all of the medical marijuana patients who have shared their stories with me. If I made a list of budtenders to thank, we would be here all day, so thank you to everyone standing behind the counter, ready to help.

And a special thank you to all of the booksellers who put this book, and all the other books, into the hands of readers. I am buying you a beer in my heart.

INDEX